Stop P

and Start Livin'

Reversing the Symptoms of
Parkinson's Disease

John C Coleman ND

MICHELLE ANDERSON PUBLISHING
MELBOURNE

First published in Australia 2005
by Michelle Anderson Publishing Pty Ltd
PO Box 6032
Chapel Street North
South Yarra 3141
Email: mapubl@bigpond.net.au
Fax: 03 9826 8552
Website: www.michelleandersonpublishing.com

Reprinted September 2006, 2009
Cover design: Deb Snibson, Modern Art Production Group
Typeset by: Midland Typesetters, Maryborough
Printed by Griffin Press

National Library of Australia Cataloguing-in-Publication data

Coleman, John.
    Stop parkin' and start livin': reversing the symptoms of
    Parkinson's disease.

    ISBN 085572 368 8.

    1. Parkinson's disease – Patients. 2. Parkinson's disease –
    Popular works. 3. Parkinson's disease – Treatment. I.

362.196833

A MESSAGE TO ALL HEALTH PRACTITIONERS

If we engage our patients with love,
approach them with humility,
speak to them with simplicity
and treat them as we would treat those we hold dearest,
then we can do no harm, and many will find their way to a
better life with our help.

John Coleman

Contents

Introduction

RETURN TO STILLNESS is a naturopathic practice, a philosophy, a way of life and a protocol for treating neurological disorders. It is this last definition which is the central focus of this book. However, we cannot separate these four definitions in reality. The protocol was developed in my clinic in Melbourne and involves both embracing a philosophy of hope and peace, and reviewing our way of life to find that peaceful strength which lies within each of us.

The RETURN TO STILLNESS protocol is not 'scientifically proven' as are some (not all) conservative Western medical treatments. In this context, 'scientifically proven' means that reproducible results are obtained when the treatment is used within a 'scientific methodology' developed in the Western world in the last sixty years or so.

The fact that there is some sort of standard by which treatments for various disorders may be measured is laudable. These standards should protect the public against practitioners or companies who seek only to make large amounts of money from selling therapies without any proof or, perhaps, any real hope of efficacy. Unfortunately, the truth is somewhat at variance to this aim. Many of our commonly used medical treatments do not qualify under the strict guidelines of 'scientific methodology'. Many drugs are allowed onto the market before we fully understand their actions, metabolic pathways, benefits, adverse effects or elimination mechanisms. For instance, in the 1980's, my son was given at least two drugs for the treatment of leukemia which were very poorly understood and yet were touted as 'good' treatment. A casual read of MIMS (a very detailed drug guide) will reveal a large number of drugs still poorly understood in one or more areas. Surgery poses different problems; we cannot construct a double blind crossover study of surgical procedures; the patient is definitely aware of whether he or she is receiving surgical treatment, and the surgeon is always aware of delivering that service. We can only look at average outcomes to see whether any surgical procedure gives benefits outweighing the risks.

Despite the doubtful 'proof' of the efficacy of some medical treatments, there are many life-saving drugs available, plus surgery and other therapies that bring great benefits to recipients. My only reason for putting forward this discussion is to clarify my position with regard to the RETURN TO STILLNESS treatment protocol. This treatment is still entirely experimental. There are no studies available to show that a large majority of people receiving this treatment recover from neurological disorders. We have not been able to construct blind or double blind studies to 'prove' the effectiveness of the treatment. We receive no funding from anyone to carry out any studies at all. There *will* be research to support the experiential hypotheses developed at RETURN TO STILLNESS, but this is in the future.

All the statements about how the RETURN TO STILLNESS treatment works, how various therapies should be used or how people do or may respond to the therapies are born of my own experience and discussion with other experienced therapists. As at this date (October 2005) my clinic appears to be the only clinic in the world fully committed to reversing the effects of the initiating trauma, and the trauma itself, as a pathway to the restoration of robust health. Many people with neurological disorders who embrace this approach come to my clinic for all their therapies. There are a significant number, however, who see other practitioners for Bowen Therapy, Flower Essences or Counselling and visit my clinic for reviews every eight to twelve weeks. There is also a growing number who undertake this journey by 'remote control' – people remote from Melbourne, both in Australia and overseas, who commence hydration and trauma recovery with instructions from Return To Stillness, and Bowen Therapy with a local therapist, without ever visiting my clinic. This is good but highlights the need for more practitioners to become involved in helping people move towards recovery from neurological disorders. As more practitioners around the world become fully at ease with this protocol, many more people will have easy access to effective treatment for neurological disorders and there is hope of this work being accepted as 'legitimate' in the future.

Many people with neurological disorders have come to my clinic since April 1998 when it first became known that I had, indeed, recovered from my own stage IV Parkinson's disease. Some have given up quickly because the work was too hard or too expensive, some because progress was too slow. Others stayed for a while and then left for similar reasons, or because their carers lost the desire to help. But many have stayed and worked hard to get well. Their progress towards recovery is a testimony to their dedication to the RETURN TO STILLNESS philosophy – **health is an individual responsibility and requires us to travel a challenging pathway, encountering obstacles to every part of our being, until we truly find that place of peace and fulfillment within ourselves and can return to stillness.**

John C Coleman

Section One

Serious Stuff

The next few chapters tell my story (very briefly), describe Parkinson's disease in conservative terms, outline my hypothesis around the cause and development of the disorder and give an insight into what it feels like to have the symptoms of Parkinson's disease. I also talk about conservative diagnostic criteria and procedures.

If you want to start on the journey to wellness quickly, and don't need to know all this stuff, flip over to SECTION TWO; I won't be insulted at all, I promise.

2

How it Began

The story of my illness and recovery is told in 'Returning To Stillness' (available through the neuro recovery foundation inc.) and 'Shaky Past' (yet to be published), with some extra details in APPENDIX 1. However, here is the very brief version.

In August 1995, after many years of slowly increasing pain, stiffness and tremor, I lost the ability to speak coherently and collapsed at my work. After visits to neurologists, a neuro-surgeon, physicians, naturopaths, osteopaths and herbalists, plus CT scans, MRI's and much general 'mucking around', I was diagnosed with Parkinson's disease (about stage IV on the Hoehn and Yahr scale) and developing Multi System Atrophy.

Because of the way I was treated during the diagnosis saga, I refused Western drug therapy (a decision supported by two very supportive surgeons I worked with at the time, and my own research into drug treatment),[1] and set out to find a way to survive day by day and, perhaps, recover some of my health. At the time, I had been studying towards a Diploma of Naturopathy for some years, so was proactive in my approach to achieving health improvement rather than control of symptoms.

In April 1998, after many wrong turns and a very challenging journey, I became symptom free. Later in 1998, I completed my Advanced Diploma of Naturopathy at the Australian College of Natural Medicine in Melbourne; it had taken 19 years of part-time study, while working full-time, to complete this goal.

Later in 1998, a gentleman was referred to me suffering from prescription-drug induced Parkinson's disease. He was unable to take Parkinson's disease medication because it would have interfered with his heart drugs. He was quite debilitated by his Parkinson's disease symptoms and unable to undertake his normal activities of lawn bowls, caring for his orchids or helping around the house. Within a few months of commencing treatment with Bowen therapy and Aqua Hydration Formulas, he was able to go back to his bowls club and resume caring for his orchids.

A woman, whom I have never met, approached me by mail and email at the end of 1998 for help with her almost total physical helplessness following years of Parkinson's disease treatment. She was just able to use a computer hesitantly and speak slowly, and was on very heavy medication. This woman chose to use the Aqua Hydration Formulas only in conjunction with her conservative Western therapies and, within four months, reported better response to medication, more mobility, increased sleep, reduced urinary frequency and a much more positive attitude towards the future.

A second gentleman came to me late in 1998 suffering from idiopathic Parkinson's disease. He was a house painter who had been forced to give up work and cease training at his football club. We commenced treatment using Bowen therapy and Aqua Hydration Formulas and, four months later, he resumed work and returned to his football club. This gentleman saw me for approximately 14 months and continued to improve in health. At one visit, he told me that there had been days without tremor, he was sleeping better and felt stronger and more agile in every way.

A story and photo in the Melbourne *Herald-Sun* newspaper in January 1999 brought phone calls and letters from all over Australia. People were desperate to find some hope of slowing, stopping or recovering from their Parkinson's disease. The more I talked to these people, the more I understood that my experience with the medical profession was not unusual. Many people volunteered that their doctors

'would not listen to me'
'treated me in an off-hand manner'
'offered no hope'
'just wanted to give me more medication'
'insisted that I take anti-depressants even though I said I wasn't depressed'.

There are many wonderful, caring doctors in the world. It seems, however, that some specialising in treatment of the aged or neuro-degenerative disorders feel that they can ride roughshod over the needs and wishes of their clients. As many people suffering from these disorders are old, debilitated, inhibited in mobility and, often, have difficulty with communication, it is easy for practitioners to assert control and impose their ideas on clients.

It quickly became apparent that I represented three benefits to people with Parkinson's disease:

1. I listened to them, and spent time with them – often 1½ hours or more;
2. I had experienced Parkinson's disease in a very severe and debilitating manifestation, so could more easily understand what they were going through;
3. I offered hope of recovery – not because I promised to cure them (I can't), but because I had recovered and

understood pretty well how I had reached my state of health.

Many people contacted me and were offered the advice described in this book. I made it clear that **there is no cure for Parkinson's disease**. However, given my own experience and that of a very few individuals around the world, **there is a way to recover**. The 'rules for recovery' from Parkinson's disease are the same now as they were in 1998 and apply to all neurological disorders.

1. There is no easy way to recover. There is no magic pill or miracle therapy that will suddenly remove all symptoms.
2. The level of symptom reversal achieved depends on disease severity, age, concomitant ailments, damage from drugs, chemicals, injury or surgery, and the level of dedication the client and their carer(s) bring to the recovery process.
3. Recovery takes a long time – at least four years and maybe much more.
4. The recovery process is multi-faceted and involves a number of therapies plus, most importantly, individual effort.
5. Full recovery can only occur if each person is treated as they deserve – ie. as a wonderful, beautiful, complex creation by the Supreme Spirit (God, the Universe, etc.) who made all things. We are all beautiful creations with unique gifts to give to this world. People with Parkinson's disease are at least as beautiful as anyone else and deserve to be treated as such.
6. Recovery requires dedicated, frustrating work on the part of the client, the carer(s) and the practitioners.

About half the people who contacted me decided that the

work demanded of them was too hard and opted out before they started. Perhaps they were not severely enough affected to warrant the task ahead; perhaps they had little to recover for; perhaps they lacked support for the struggle. Whatever the reason, they decided that the certainty of continued medication and ultimate degeneration into helplessness was preferable to the uncertainty of a struggle to recover with only one claim of complete recovery (me). I don't blame them for that, but I am saddened when I see others progressing so well toward recovery and understand how far towards health those who dropped out could be.

Others started the process and worked hard, then dropped out after a few months or a year. Usually the reason given was lack of progress, yet everyone who dropped out had made progress. Why couldn't they see this? Often because they failed to keep diaries or notes on their feelings and physical condition over time. Therefore, when they felt 'bad' after a year's work, they had no reference point from the past to see that, in reality, their 'bad feeling' today was so much better than their 'bad feeling' a few months ago. Sometimes it was their carer (spouse/child/sibling) who just got tired of running around and spending money on a sick person and decided that progress was not fast enough. This was tragic after so much hard work and good progress.

There are many people, however, who have continued to struggle on despite their frustration and impatience. They are now being rewarded with improving health and, eventually, some will fully recover from their symptoms of Parkinson's disease as I did.

Wild Medicine, manufacturers of the Aqua Hydration Formulas, undertook some research testing during 2001 to gain a better understanding of the recovery process. I was a participant in these tests.

While the findings are complex, some basic facts became clear. Hydration, using the Aqua Hydration Formulas, accounted for about 60% of my physical recovery. Bowen Therapy added another 25% to the journey. Therefore, the combination of Aqua Hydration Formulas and Bowen Therapy is the most powerful part of the physical recovery process. However, these therapies must be accompanied by dedication and committed effort on the part of each person suffering from Parkinson's disease and their carers. Without this dedication and determination to be well, we cannot recover.

Another most interesting finding from this research was that Parkinson's disease seems to involve much more than just a deficiency of dopamine. Many other neurotransmitters are deficient. Therefore it is likely that other neurological disorders are also more complex than is thought at the moment.

The implication of this finding is that we cannot concentrate on just replacing one chemical, or repairing one tiny section of brain. We must focus on a total restoration of brain tissue and brain function, as well as emotional and spiritual development, to achieve full recovery.

As with all illness, we have a choice to resign ourselves to continuing illness, or recognise our great strength and move towards health with determination and faith, making use of all available resources.

People with 'incurable' diseases are getting well! Some take a very long time – four years or more. Some move more quickly. We don't understand all the reasons for this difference, or why some just seem to slip further down the degenerative slope despite all our efforts. What we do observe, however, is that all those who make significant progress in improving their health set out to find a centre of peace within themselves, begin to believe that they are loved and worth loving, and understand that the most important things in life are their beautiful spiritual being, love of and for themselves, love for those close to them, their physical health, and material possessions sufficient to allow them to live in reasonable comfort – in that order.

It may be many years before we really understand the recovery process, but we do know that people have unequivocally recovered from Parkinson's disease, Multiple Sclerosis, a variety of auto-immune disorders, Fibromyalgia (and Polymyalgia), and more are contacting us each month with their stories of recovery. Through the neuro recovery foundation inc. and my own work, we will continue to spread the knowledge that there are no incurable diseases, just incurable people. We now know that 'cure' is just a word, recovery *is* possible.

3

Parkinson's Disease –
A Conservative View

You might want to skip this section as it explores general, con-
servative information about Parkinson's disease that is available
from Parkinson's support groups and associations, and many
websites. However, most of your doctors base their understand-
ing and treatment on the basic information included here, so
you may be interested in browsing through it.

The World Health Organisation estimates that there are
about four million people worldwide with Parkinson's
disease. According to The National Parkinson Foundation
website (www.parkinson.org), about 1.5 million Americans
have been diagnosed with Parkinson's disease, while over
60,000 are newly diagnosed each year. About 15% of those
diagnosed are under 50 years of age. The University of
Birmingham's Department of Clinical Neurosciences suggests that '1–2% of the elderly' in UK develop Parkinson's
disease. Parkinson's disease affects an estimated one percent
of Australians in the 75–80 year age group[12] and a total of
20,000 to 40,000 Australians in all age groups (there are no
official statistics available).

The severity of the disease varies from mild, untreated
symptoms (stages 0 to I) to debilitating symptoms necessitating full-time care (stage V). Idiopathic Parkinson's disease

is primarily a problem associated with advancing age, however, there are significant numbers of early-onset Parkinson's disease sufferers, some as young as in their twenties. Non-idiopathic, or secondary Parkinson's disease has no age barriers but is a much less common condition.

Parkinson's disease (also known as Parkinson's Syndrome, Parkinsonism, Paralysis Agitans and Shaking Palsy) is a chronic, progressive Central Nervous System disorder characterised by slowness and poverty of purposeful movement, muscular rigidity and tremor.[2] Parkinsonism is essentially a set of symptoms rather than a disease as pathological changes can only be surveyed post mortem.

A variant, or extension of Parkinsonism is Multi System Atrophy (MSA, Multiple System Atrophy,[3,4] idiopathic orthostatic hypotension, Shy-Drager syndrome).[3,5] Often exhibited by boxers, this differs from classical Parkinson's disease in the type and extent of physical symptoms in that the gait tends to be wider and less festinating, an intention tremor often either replaces, or is in addition to, the resting tremor, and motor dysfunction is often more apparent. However, the MSA patient may present with typically Parkinsonian symptoms and needs to be observed carefully at examination before confirming diagnosis. MSA may occur as a result of a single, dramatic cerebral trauma or repeated trauma to the head as sustained by boxers ('punch-drunk' syndrome), or abused wives and children.[4]

Parkinson's disease was first described in detail by James Parkinson in 1817 in his essay on the Shaking Palsy, however, some researchers believe it to be a condition as old as man in that it is essentially a condition of cell death during the ageing process. This view is not necessarily universal as there is a developing body of thought linking Parkinson's disease with pollution and heavy metal toxicity.[5,6] Free radical damage is also postulated as a possible cause, again linked to our polluted, nutritionally poor lifestyle.[6] As you will see in a later chapter, I have posed a serious hypothesis around the cause and development of Parkinson's disease that is now being supported by neurological research around the world.[13]

Pathologically, Parkinson's disease is characterised by aggregation of melanin-containing nerve cells and varying degrees of cell loss with reactive gliosis in the substantia nigra and locus caeruleus of the basal ganglia, with a high population of Lewy bodies.[7] The biochemical result is a decrease of dopamine in the caudate nucleus and putamen. Dopamine is an inhibitory neurotransmitter and balances the excitatory function of acetylcholine in the caudate and putamen basal ganglia.[8,9] Any loss of dopaminergic cells provides a relative excess of cholinergic activity resulting in hypertonia (the Parkinsonian tremor and rigidity) and akinesia.[8,10]

Again I must emphasise that this is a very conservative view and is at odds with my experience showing deficiencies in a large number of neurotransmitters.

The classical manifestations of Parkinson's disease are resting tremor, muscle rigidity and akinesia (lack of normal movement). These may develop alone or in combination but, as the disease progresses, all will be present to some degree. The symptoms usually develop asymmetrically but eventually become truly bilateral, although there may still be asymmetry about the severity of some symptoms. Postural abnormalities, autonomic-neuroendocrine symptoms and, sometimes, dementia are also part of the syndrome.[8,9] These later symptoms may also be the result of long-term ingestion of drugs used to control Parkinsonian symptoms.[1]

The pathophysiology of Parkinson's disease post mortem shows a progressive reduction in the number and activity of nigrostriatal dopamine neurones and a massive reduction in striatal dopamine content.[11] However, in most cases, the cause of these changes is still a matter for conjecture.

Idiopathic Parkinson's Disease

The disease does not show any hereditary pattern or strong familial tendency, nor any particular population patterns.[5,8] Epidemiological studies have suggested vascular, viral and metabolic factors as possible causes[8] but there is, as yet, no consensus on any one or combination of these factors as a definitive cause. One hypothesis is that age predisposes the nigrostriatal pathway to damage by viruses or toxins.[8] However, this begs the question of why only one percent of the ageing population[12] develops this disease when rationality would suggest that all those who age with exposure to the same viruses or toxins would display some or all Parkinsonian symptoms before death.

While there is a significant amount of research into methods of controlling Parkinsonian symptoms, and into trying to understand the processes involved during the development of Parkinson's disease, little is yet known by conservative scientists about likely causes.

From a naturopathic point of view, our bio-individuality probably provides the answer. We all age, but the rate of ageing and the way we express the ageing process varies from individual to individual. Factors influencing the way we age include genetic inheritance, environment, nutrition, contact with toxins, our spiritual pathway and, particularly, significant experiences during childhood.[13] There is much to be learned about the metaphysical meaning of Parkinson's disease symptoms, and part of my research is devoted to trying to understand what series of physical or emotional events might persuade a person to display their 'dis-ease' as Parkinsonian symptoms.

Drug induced Parkinson's Disease

Parkinsonian symptoms are most commonly caused by the **Phenothiazines, haloperidol and reserpine.**[5]

The *Phenothiazines* are commonly used antipsychotic drugs and include Chlorpromozine, Promazine, Triflupromazine, Mesoridazine, Piperacetazine, Thioridazine, Acetophenazine, Butaperazine, Carphenazine, Fluphenazine, Perphenazine, Prochlorperazine, Trifluperazine, Methotrimeprazine, Pericyazine, Piperazine and Pipothiazine. These drugs have a number of moderate to severe side effects and are all catecholamine blockers (noradrenaline and dopamine); it is this action which causes Parkinsonian symptoms (akathisia, tremor and rigidity). High doses of Phenothiazines given over a long period may cause irreversible tardive dyskinesia which is easily confused with idiopathic Parkinson's disease symptoms.[5,14] The use of Levodopa in individuals suffering from Phenothiazine induced Parkinsonism is ineffective and may, in fact, exacerbate the symptoms.

Haloperidol is a Butyrophone derivative and is used to control behavioural dysfunction in all age groups. Haloperidol blocks dopamine receptors in the Central Nervous System. Side effects vary with age and sex and Parkinsonian symptoms are most common in the elderly, although middle-aged patients may develop akathisia which can be confused with a Parkinsonian tremor. Haloperidol diminishes the effect of Levodopa and aggravates Parkinson's disease in patients using Levodopa therapy.[5]

Reserpine is a Rauwolfia alkaloid used as an antipsychotic drug in the past, but rarely prescribed now. It is occasionally used as a hypotensive drug. Reserpine exacerbates the symptoms of Parkinson's disease.[5,14]

The 'designer drug' **MPTP** (methylphenyl-tetrahydro-pyridine) and heart drugs such as **verapamil** and **amiodarone** have been implicated in causing or exacerbating Parkinson's disease. **Non-steroidal anti-inflammatory drugs (NSAID's)** such as **Naproxen** may also aggravate Parkinson's disease.[15] Parkinsonism has been commonly reported after using **Calcium-Channel Blockers** such as **flumarizine** and **cinnarizine**. Symptoms abated rapidly when medication was withdrawn, except in a few patients who still displayed Parkinsonian symptoms 18 months after withdrawal of medication.[16]

Drug induced Parkinson's disease is normally reversible except as noted above.[5,8]

Toxicity induced Parkinson's Disease

Carbon Monoxide and **Manganese** poisoning may cause Parkinson's disease.[5] With increasing air pollution in our cities, and heavy metal pollution in our food chain, toxicity induced Parkinson's disease may become more common.

Studies around the world have indicated a relationship between excessive **iron** (and other heavy metals) and Parkinsonism. In the presence of a high concentration of iron, dopamine can auto-oxidise to form free radicals and damage the basal ganglia.[6]

Other causes of Parkinson's Disease

Bilateral infarcts of the basal ganglia, hydrocephalus, tumours near the basal ganglia and cerebral trauma may also cause the syndrome.[5,8] Post-encephalitic Parkinsonism commonly followed the 1919–1924 pandemic of encephalitis lethargica; this is now very rare.[5]

A rare form of inherited Parkinson's disease, **autosomal recessive juvenile parkinsonism (AR-JP)** is caused by a mutated gene recently discovered by scientists at the Keio University School of Medicine in Tokyo. There may be some link between this mutated gene and idiopathic Parkinson's disease, but this is, as yet, uncertain.[17]

Stages of Parkinson's Disease

The stages of the syndrome used above and throughout this book are assessed on the **Hoehn and Yahr Scale.**[18]

- STAGE 0 = no clinically discernible syndrome
- STAGE I = syndrome is unilateral
- STAGE II = bilateral syndrome without balance impairment
- STAGE III = syndrome impairs balance or walking
- STAGE IV = syndrome markedly impairs balance or walking
- STAGE V = syndrome results in complete immobility

While this scale is extremely limited in the scope of symptoms it references, it is useful in enabling a uniform classification of disease severity where required. A more complete assessment of the progress of Parkinson's disease can be obtained using the Unified Parkinson's Disease Rating Scale (UPDRS) or similar measures.

4

What About Stress?

Since 1998, I have seen hundreds of people diagnosed with Parkinson's disease by neurologists, and treated with normal Western drugs. In each case, I have taken the most thorough history possible, including details of conception and birth, childhood, and relationships with parents and siblings. At first, this was simply an exercise in finding out as much as I could about each person so that I could understand their responses, the best way to approach challenges, and how I could relate to them in the best way. By the end of 2000, I had noticed a pattern of life history that first intrigued me, then blossomed as a revelation, and helped me understand more about my own disease process and recovery.

Following my collapse in August 1995, I spent four weeks at home on sick leave, trying to find ways to survive alone. My first response was hopelessness, apathy and unbearable weariness. Then I became angry as I, for some reason, began to review my childhood and family relationships. There is no doubt that my early life was tough, as it was for my whole family then. My father was serving in the air force (it was 1943 and he was posted to Darwin). My mother lived in a primitive house with a single water tap, outside toilet and no sewerage. Money and food were scarce, and she had two children to care for, as well as being pregnant with me. I have no doubt that her very high stress levels affected me as I developed in her womb.[13]

A 'normal' birth was followed by poor nutrition, lack of

proper attention, illness and abuse in a variety of guises over about ten years. At about nine years old, I was so worn down by my family life that I tried to take my own life. Fortunately, I did not succeed or I would have missed the best time of my life.

My life review, during the first four weeks of Parkinson's disease, brought me to the conclusion that my start in life had something to do with my illness, but I did not then understand the real connection.[13,19]

Finding a pattern of unresolved stress or trauma in the lives of all those diagnosed with Parkinson's disease who came to my clinic, set me off on a search for answers. Could unresolved stress prepare our bodies for the expression of Parkinson's disease symptoms?[13,19] So I began studying the chemical processes that occur in trauma and stress, and the long-term effects of those chemicals when they remain at an abnormal level over long periods.[13,19]

The physiology of stress

There is excellent research into genetic factors and the physiological processes that take place during the development of Parkinson's disease. It seems to me, however, that most research looks at factors too close in time to diagnosis. While family history is considered and either held as a risk factor, or discounted as such, the full life and health history of the patient is rarely taken or considered important.

Non-medical therapists I have spoken to over the past few years seem to share the view of conservative science that neurological disorders develop over six to ten years and, in most cases of Parkinson's disease, there are few lifestyle factors involved.

I do not have the benefit of years of very expensive research and, therefore, can only present my views as hypotheses, yet to be proven or disproved under rigorous examination. It is reassuring to read that neuro scientists are now considering experiences in early life as a causative or exacerbating factor in chronic and degenerative disease.[13,19] Perhaps stating my hypotheses will encourage someone to come forward with funding for more rigorous research.

One factor stands out as a common denominator among all my patients with Parkinson's disease. Each person has experienced high stress or trauma at some stage during their first fifteen years. Most had this experience during their first ten years. Many of the traumas are obvious – abuse of various types, loss of a parent or sibling, life-threatening disease or accident. Some are not so obvious. For instance, a woman who was implicitly blamed by her father for her mother's miscarriage; a woman adopted into a loving family after nine months of bonding to her birth mother; a man whose father was a workaholic and was not around for any of his son's activities, or present to develop a relationship.

Sometimes it is simply being born at a time or in a place that is traumatic. For instance those born in Europe just before or during WWII, or in Eastern Europe during the Soviet occupation. Their families lived in fear and uncertainty; babies were conceived and born into traumatic circumstances. For those predisposed to Parkinson's disease, this may be the initiating stress overload.

Stress can be good for us as it motivates us to activity, and provides the physiological resources for that activity. Without some level of stress, we would not get out of bed in the morning.[13,19]

Trauma need not be physically damaging if it is treated and resolved healthily and holistically.[13] But this is rare in the sorts of trauma mentioned above.

Prolonged stress and unresolved trauma trigger our body

into continuous stress reactions that, over a long time, become damaging.[13,19]

The initial physiological reaction to any type of significant stress or trauma is the 'flight or fight' response. Simply put, the process is this:

- The adrenal glands have two major parts, the *medulla* and **cortex**
- Excretion of adrenal *medullary hormones* is directly triggered by stress and trauma
- Stress and trauma stimulate the **hypothalamus** to release Corticotropin-releasing Hormone (CRH)
- CRH stimulates the release of Adrenocorticotropic Hormone (ACTH) from the Pituitary Gland
- ACTH regulates excretions from the **adrenal cortex**.

Hormones released by the adrenals are:

MEDULLA (amino acid derivative)	Adrenaline (plus small amounts of nor adrenaline)
CORTEX (steroids)	Mineralocorticoids (aldosterone) Glucocorticoids (cortisol) Adrenal androgens (testosterone)

Effects of adrenal hormones:

Adrenaline
- Increases blood glucose by activating cyclic AMP
- Increases glycogen breakdown (decreases reserves)
- Increases intracellular metabolism of glucose in skeletal muscles (ready for action)
- Increases breakdown of fats in adipose (fatty) tissue
- Increases heart rate

- Increases force of heart contraction
- Constricts blood vessels in skin, kidneys, gastrointestinal tract and other organs not needed for fight/flight
- Dilates blood vessels in skeletal and cardiac muscle

Aldosterone
- Increases rate of sodium reabsorption in kidneys
  - Increased plasma sodium
  - Increased water reabsorption (that can lead to oedema)
  - Increased blood volume (that can lead to hypertension)
- Increases potassium excretion (lower plasma potassium)
- Increases hydrogen ion excretion (leading to acidic urine, increased metabolic pH-alkalosis)
- Changes in sodium/potassium balance can affect cellular hydration, cell membrane function and transport to and from cells

Cortisol
- Increases catabolism of fats
- Decreases glucose and amino acid uptake in skeletal muscles
- Increases glucose synthesis from amino acids in the liver leading to increased blood glucose
- Increases protein degradation (leading to muscle weakness/ atrophy, osteoporosis)
- Decreases inflammatory response by decreasing number of white cells and the expression of inflammatory chemicals (leading to a depressed immune system)

Testosterone *(indirect and mainly in women)*
- Increases pubic and axillary hair
- Increases sexual drive (but may reduce potency)

Short-term stress is a normal part of life. We need it for motivation, and we need the physiological responses to stress in order to survive. Our forebears faced immediate dangers and stimuli every day – for instance, they needed to chase down prey, or run away from predators, or fight enemies to protect their territory or families.

In all these cases, the stress was resolved quite quickly – they won or lost, caught the prey or waited until the next day, got away or got eaten.[13]

We have negative feedback systems to adjust levels of adrenal hormones so they do not become damaging. However, **stress can override these negative feedback systems** so that we go on hyper-producing these chemicals.[13] Evolution decided that all stress was necessary, so our body was the best judge of whether we needed adrenal hormones or not. Evolution didn't bargain on the long-term stresses of Western society. Furthermore, Western society has developed so quickly that our evolution processes can't keep up. Our physiological ability to cope with modern stresses has lagged way behind the development of those stressors.[13]

Many stresses in this society are not resolved, and many traumas go unrecognised.[13] We live surrounded by noise, pollution, busy-ness and poisons. Child abuse is the world's best-kept secret; family breakdown is seen as traumatic for the partners, but not necessarily for the children; the loss of a sibling or grandparent or friend is often borne in silence by the young in our society.

Prolonged and unresolved stress or trauma can result in:

Increased plasma sodium
Decreased plasma potassium
Cellular dehydration

Reprogramming of the hypothalamus
Chronic heart stress and eventual failure
Alkalosis (often treated with antacids!)
Hypertension
Weak skeletal muscles
Acidic urine
Hyperglycemia leading to diabetes mellitus
Deficient immune system
Muscle atrophy
General weakness and debility
Osteoporosis
Weak capillaries
Thin skin that bruises easily
Impaired wound healing
Inappropriate fat distribution (face, neck, abdomen)
Mood swings (euphoria and/or depression)

In women

Hirsutism
Increased sex drive
Diminished breast size
Menstrual irregularities

People facing prolonged, unresolved stress or trauma will respond in different ways, possibly dictated by their genetic inheritance and/or environment. Some will develop heart disease, cancer, arthritis, diabetes, skin disorders, depression or other psychological disorders, gastric ulcers or inappropriate behaviour such as substance addictions, addictive gambling or violent behaviour.[13,19]

Some will develop Parkinson's disease. The reprogramming of the hypothalamus and cellular dehydration, as well as many of the other effects shown above, allow some brain cells to become damaged or inactive, or even die, over many years, ultimately resulting in the expression of Parkinson's disease symptoms.

Stress/trauma is not necessarily the 'cause' of Parkinson's disease, but can begin the slow degeneration that leads to cell fragility and damage.[13,19] All those I see also have a history of stress triggers throughout life, and a high degree of imposed responsibility for others. This is also a factor in disease development, and I will discuss this in a later chapter.

Once we recognise that our Parkinson's disease is not our fault, and there is a logical development process, we can create strategies to reverse the process and, perhaps, recover.

Is it enough to see Parkinson's as a process or a disease?

People diagnosed with Parkinson's disease are, first and foremost, people. We are individuals with life experiences, relationships, ambitions, successes and failures. Our disorder is a part of the amazing, complex adventure that is our individual life, and cannot be separated from that context if we are to find our way to robust health.

Western medicine seeks to define us by a disease – *you have Parkinson's disease, or Multi System Atrophy or Progressive Supranuclear Palsy* – and confirms this with standard tests, scans and medication responses. Reducing us to a disease state enables mechanistic treatment within a limited understanding of physiological processes.

Many complementary therapists try to define us as organ system functions – *your liver needs work, your parathyroid is sluggish and your gut is really bad* – as if we can be reduced to the sum of our parts. A few see beyond the disorder and help to release us from the prison of our experience.

When we develop Parkinson's disease symptoms, we are

already vastly experienced in our life; we have spent years, one way or another, developing our life path, building knowledge unique to us, creating a wonderful, complex, unique being that has never been on this planet before, and never will be here again. Our disorder has developed in a unique way, and so cannot be defined or described with generalist or reductionist language. As practitioners, we need to develop skills and a language that relates to each individual, and creates a bond of trust and understanding that allows our patient to fully express the spiritual, emotional, intellectual and physical interactions that have led them, uniquely, to display their particular symptoms. It is only within this environment of spiritual interaction that we, as practitioners, can begin to understand how best to support each person's journey to wellness.

Doctors and, especially, specialists such as neurologists, are placed in an invidious position when judging the health of their patients and recommending treatment. Their training does not allow for any definition or judgment other than an artificially created 'scientific methodology', developed mainly during the twentieth century, that seeks to reduce each person, disease or process to it's individual parts, and not look beyond that. So we see patients diagnosed with Parkinson's disease, hypertension, heart disease, diabetes mellitus and osteoarthritis, treated by five or six different specialists all looking only at their limited area of expertise and prescribing treatment accordingly. In the rigmarole of appointments, referrals, tests, scans, examinations and form filling, the patients lose their right to exist as an individual, and become a 'case' for each practitioner, to be defined by data, treated by statistical outcome and lost in the cauldron of mechanistic medicine.

We have to do better. As individual patients, we deserve practitioners who are brave enough to listen to what we say, to observe our gestures and facial expressions indicating our deepest feelings, inexpressible in words. We deserve practitioners who will give time and energy to developing a bond and teamwork that has nothing to do with tests, examinations, scans, laboratory research, statistics or data; practitioners who have the courage and patience to communicate with us at a spiritual level, so that we can find our true being hidden behind the prison bars of physical disease.

It is not enough to say that only those who experience disease can truly understand disease. Health practitioners cannot be fortunate enough to experience every disease we treat and, as we well know, each individual experiences each disorder in a unique way. We can, however, develop observational and communication skills that allow us to reach a much closer understanding of what each patient is experiencing in *their* terms. We can listen without judging, observe without pre-empting our observations, and develop a picture of each individual in the context of *their* life experience, values, culture, expectations and ambitions.

Seeking health is not a war. We speak about *fighting disease, acceptable risks, statistical success rates.* These have nothing to do with health. Robust health is to be welcomed, nurtured, treated with love and kindness. We can seek health, embrace it, welcome it into our lives and be joyful at its appearance.

As practitioners, we can be joyful with our patients when there is a move towards health, encouraging and supportive when the journey seems hard, and provide strategies, and a language, that brings power into our patients' lives and enables them to continue in their joyous embrace of robustness.

Only when we develop a language and a manner that allows the empowerment of each patient on their unique road to health will we be truly able to assist in recovery from ostensibly incurable disorders.

5

But What Does it Feel Like?
– Living Behind the Mask

There are many physical and emotional states surrounding the onset and development of Parkinson's disease. Most are poorly understood except by those suffering from the disease. While each individual will walk their own particular journey, many of our experiences are shared to a great degree.

At diagnosis, we all experience fear. Whether our diagnosis has been sudden or protracted, the words 'you have Parkinson's disease' bring fear because we 'know' it is incurable, and we don't really know what is going to happen.

The onset of symptoms can bring embarrassment, frustration, pain and fatigue. Most people find their tremor embarrassing; especially as it begins to inhibit normal actions such as drinking or eating. Some become isolated, finding the embarrassment too great to enable them to mix in public. As we slow down and lose coordination, we become frustrated. We can no longer do some of the enjoyable things we could just a short while ago. Some may have to modify their work, or even give up work altogether. We start to drop and break precious items; our walk becomes slower and less rhythmical; it takes longer to carry out simple tasks like dressing, cleaning, cooking, getting into the car, frustrating our partners or friends as well as ourselves. Constipation and incontinence are both embarrassing and frustrating, as is the dribbling experienced by many.

Pain is not experienced by everyone, but when it is, it can vary from intermittent cramping to constant, nagging, debilitating agony. Fatigue is constant; we all suffer from it to some degree. In the early stages of our disorder, we may just get a little more tired in the afternoon and find it hard to stay awake in front of television at night. As the disease progresses, we begin to feel exhausted throughout the day, often finding that every movement requires enormous effort, as if walking against a chest-high opposing current. Yet this is not just a physical tiredness; it is as if our spirit is exhausted from the effort of existence, and can find no relief in sleep, nourishment, or even prayer.

The predominant feeling with Parkinson's disease is an increasing isolation from the rest of the world as our activities become more laboured, our face loses the ability to express emotion, we become too tired to assert ourselves and we sense our lives slipping away. Often we feel as if there is a glass wall around us separating us from those we love or need to relate to. We call, scream, plead for recognition and understanding, but nobody hears through the glass. We try to give signals, but our body either won't move or moves abnormally, so those around us see only the physical, and cannot hear our spiritual agony.

People confined to wheelchairs – paraplegics and quadriplegics for instance – have spoken to me about being treated 'as if they are not there' or intellectually handicapped. Many with Parkinson's disease have similar experiences. They may be ignored in shops, spoken to as if they are young children, or shouted at as if deaf. A member of my family visited me when I was first diagnosed, and shouted at me in childish sentences as if my stammer and tremor were the result of intellectual retardation. My replies were ignored.

It is this sort of treatment that makes us nervous, or even

fearful, of mixing in normal society. Our anxiety inevitably increases our symptoms when we do venture out, so we drop things, spill food and drink or become incontinent even though we are managing very well in the safe environment of our home.

Living behind the mask of Parkinson's disease is isolating, frightening, frustrating, debilitating, exhausting and depressing. We long to reach out with our warmth and excitement, but our mask of disease prevents us. We turn inwards and become obsessed with trivia or our condition. We appear sullen and disinterested, but that is just our mask. We cry for help, but are told we can't be helped. We long for energy and vitality, but are told we must live with crumbling, aching bodies. We are treated with anti-depressant drugs, yet the cause of our depressed emotions, our lack of hope, is not addressed.

I have experienced two terrifying events in my life. One was telling my eleven-year-old son that he was going to die. The other was walking through the dark valley of Parkinson's disease. The first event lasted two hours, the second three years. I no longer know which was the more difficult.

When you meet someone with Parkinson's disease, remember that they are fragile, anxious, desperate and, until recently, have been given no hope. Treat them as delicate buds about to bloom. With hope, help and motivation, **we can recover** from Parkinson's disease.

6

Diagnosis

When fully developed, Parkinson's disease is unmistakable; the typical features of fixed expression, stooped posture, festinating walk, slow movement and resting tremor distinguish it from other disorders.[5,9] At post-mortem, diagnosis is again relatively easy with evidence of cell destruction in the substantia nigra and the presence of Lewy bodies.[3]

During early development, however, diagnosis is often difficult and depends on the rate and symmetry with which symptoms appear, and the exclusion of other likely causes for the symptoms.[3,5,9]

There is no universally accepted criteria for the diagnosis of Parkinson's disease. However, Larsen, Dupont and Tandberg have proposed a set of criteria to allow diagnosis with various levels of confidence.[3] Under this proposal, to be definitely diagnosed with Idiopathic Parkinson's disease, a patient must display the following:

1. The presence of at least two of the following three symptoms:
   a) resting tremor
   b) rigidity
   c) postural abnormality.
2. Unilateral onset of symptoms and asymmetrical development.
3. Good to excellent response to dopamine agonist drugs or l'dopa drugs.

4. At the onset of the disease, absence of significant changes on CT or MRI other than mild diffuse cortical atrophy or mild hypertense periventricular foci on MRI. Absence of clinical exclusion criteria like dementia, pyramidal and cerebellar signs and autonomic failure which may indicate another neurodegenerative disorder. Absence of environmental factors like drugs and toxic substances or a history of encephalitis that may cause a symptomatic Parkinsonism.

While these criteria serve to rationalise clinical diagnosis of Parkinson's disease, the early stages of disease development is insidious and can often be mistaken for general malaise, depression, stress or a 'natural' ageing process.

The medical model seeks to precisely classify patients as definitely Parkinson's disease, probable Parkinson's disease, or definitely not Parkinson's disease. However, like most disease processes, Parkinson's disease does not necessarily adhere to a particular man-made model. Any or all of the symptoms listed below may be displayed by those with Parkinson's disease and, while some more typically appear early in development, the total symptom picture should be considered before a diagnosis is made or rejected.

Symptoms[3,4,5,8,9,12]

1. **Resting tremor** usually beginning in one hand or finger and often displaying a 'pill-rolling' characteristic. The tremor may, however, begin in the lips or head and may be more apparent when tired, embarrassed or confused. Tremor is often apparent in lightly closed eyelids.
2. **Bradykinesia** (slow movements or difficulty initiating movement), sometimes variable in that patients may carry out complex tasks as usual when motivated by

interest or goal achievement, but slow down when the motivation ceases. This is especially apparent in voluntary movement carried out by small muscle groups. Bradykinesia may also be exacerbated by emotional stress.

3. **Stooped posture**, often asymmetrical, as if the centre of balance had moved forward and to one side. Posture may become unstable with unexplained falls or 'walking into things'.

4. **Muscle rigidity** caused by hypertonia (muscles remaining in a contracted state) involving opposing muscle groups. This may manifest in hypertonic muscle groups apparent on palpation, or in 'cogwheel' jerking when moving limbs or the head instead of smooth, flowing movements. However, movements may just become stiff (especially passive movement) as hypertonic muscles resist. Grasping may be inhibited and patients may drop items or be unable to catch or lift things.

5. **Fixed facial expression**. Hypertonic muscles cause the face to form into a more or less rigid mask showing little animation. Under challenge, especially pleasurable challenge, response may occur with some delay. The facial rigidity is likely to develop asymmetrically. The mouth may be slightly open and some unchecked drooling from the corners may occur. The eyes blink infrequently and appear to stare, moving only slowly to follow points of interest.

6. **Walk.** The patient may 'drag' one leg, or find it difficult to start walking but walk well once started, or walk more slowly than previously, or display the typical festinating walk associated with Parkinson's disease. When the festinating walk develops, the patient begins to stride normally but the steps become shorter and quicker and

the patient leans forward as if trying to catch up with their own centre of balance. They may break into a shuffling, uncontrollable trot as if walking down a very steep slope without support. The arms may be held away from the body and bent at the elbow as if to maintain balance.

7. **'Freezing'.** The patient may find it difficult to begin tasks other than walking. For example, they may stand in front of a cupboard door without being able to grasp the handle and open it, or they may not be able to rise from a chair. Turning corners when walking may be very difficult and require the patient to come to a complete stop, then undertake some 'tricks' to commence the new task of turning.

8. **Speech** may become slurred, slow, soft, garbled, or fluctuate between all these. In normal circumstances there may be only a progressive slowness of speech apparent with, perhaps, a little reduction in normal volume and/or change in timbre. Under stress, or with fatigue, the speech may become slurred (as if drunk or following a stroke) or completely incoherent even though thought processes remain coherent and quick.

9. **Diminished muscle strength** as a result of hypertonicity, bradykinesia, freezing and a diminished 'nerve message' supply to the muscles. Over time, as activity reduces, muscles may display a reduction in bulk and/or atrophy.

10. **Difficulty with bed mobility.** It may be difficult to turn in bed because of rigidity, or the patient may not be able to recruit the muscles required to turn even though they know what they want to do.

11. **Fatigue.** Unexplained fatigue, often extreme, may cause confusion in diagnosis as it mimics the fatigue in Chronic Fatigue Syndrome, Clinical Depression, Hypoglycemia and similar syndromes.

12. **Difficulty in performing simultaneous tasks** which are otherwise uncomplicated (eg. sitting on the edge of the bed with arms outstretched and eyes closed).

13. **Orthostatic hypotension** may be an indication that neck muscle rigidity is causing a reduction of blood flow to the brain.

14. **Urinary frequency or incontinence or urinary retention** without prostatic changes or any sign of urinary tract infection.

15. **Muscle and bone pain** caused by hypertonicity and secondary joint changes. Pain may range from a mild, dull ache, to extreme cramping pain without apparent cause and be difficult to control.

16. **Depression.** It is a matter of contention as to whether depression is a symptom of Parkinson's disease, or the other symptoms of·Parkinson's disease cause the patient to become depressed about their condition and prognosis. However, Parkinsonian patients are often depressed. Standard treatment is with anti-depressants which may exacerbate Parkinsonian symptoms and confuse the source of the depression.[1] Typical Parkinsonian symptoms such as fixed expression, slurred speech, bradykinesia, clumsiness and drooling are humiliating for the patient and often lead others to treat patients as if they are intellectually or physically deficient. Treatment as 'a retard' added to normal anxiety about their condition can lead to quite severe depression.[20]

17. **Autonomic nervous system** depression may cause subtle changes early in development, with more obvious changes apparent as the disease progresses. These changes may include respiratory or heart rate fluctuations, reduced oxygen saturation, reduced appetite and constipation caused by reduced feedback mechanism.

18. **Neuroendocrine symptoms** such as inappropriate diaphoresis (sweating), gastric retention, oily skin with seborrheic dermatitis along the hairline and in the chin or nasal creases.

19. **Reduction in libido and/or impotence** is common. Fatigue is obviously a factor here, but often situations normally arousing response will fail to do so some or all of the time. This is usually very embarrassing and frustrating for the patient as they have no logical explanation for their lack of response. Again, 'the mind and spirit are more than willing but the body says no!'

The picture presented by a Parkinsonian patient early in the development of the disease is rarely, if ever, clear-cut. Symptoms develop slowly and insidiously, often causing the patient to blame themselves for becoming clumsy, or slowing down with age. Even when seeking diagnosis, patients will continue to blame themselves for some of the symptoms, be too embarrassed to tell of some (eg. incontinence, impotence) and become confused over time and relative progress of symptoms. Definitive diagnosis requires time, patience and empathy on the part of health practitioners involved in the process.

Section Two

Serious Stuff, But Really Important

In this section, I suggest some helpful ways to handle diagnosis, and how you can begin to help yourself.

If we are to achieve truly good health, we must take the major role in creating that good health. We cannot rely on doctors, naturopaths, counsellors or other therapists to do it for us.

We are the expert on our health.

We are the most powerful therapist we have.

We have, within us, the ability to heal any wound or illness if we choose to grasp that ability and work hard with it.

In this section, I talk about some of the activities, life changes and philosophies you can embrace to help yourself. You may find many more; follow those with enthusiasm also.

If you do nothing more than follow these suggestions you will make a profound improvement to your lfe.

This is the most important section, so if you read nothing else read this section twice.

7

So You've Just Been Diagnosed With Parkinson's Disease

'You have Parkinson's disease' are words that can sound like a death sentence when delivered by a practitioner who is not sensitive to our needs. Most practitioners have never experienced the ravages this disorder can cause, and so make judgements based on technical data, without much appreciation or understanding of the deep emotional and spiritual issues involved.

Our diagnosis often makes us feel that we have lost control of our life, and can do nothing about it. We feel that we are now in the hands of 'experts', must obey every instruction given to us, and have no power to help ourselves.

Wrong! We can help ourselves. We can take control of our life and chart our own course towards the health we desire.

1. *Don't panic*. Parkinson's disease is a slow-moving disorder that won't kill you. All those dreadful symptoms and eventualities you may have been told about are a long way off, and can be delayed or prevented. You have lots of time to look at options, make choices, talk to many people and gather as much information as you want.[21]
2. *Keep living your life to the full*. Don't give up work or hobbies and shut yourself away. The best medicine for

Parkinson's disease is laughter, joy, love and fulfilling activity.

3. *Find a neurologist who will talk to you simply and calmly*, give you lots of easy-to-understand information, and spend as much time with you as you need. If the neurologist who gave you the diagnosis does not fit these criteria, find another. You don't have to stay with any doctor or specialist who does not meet your needs.[21]

4. If you have problems finding a suitable neurologist, *seek out other people* with Neurological Disorders (Parkinson's Disease, Multiple Sclerosis, Motor Neurone Disorder) and ask them how they relate to their neurologist. It is sometimes a good idea to find a neurologist who isn't as busy as the 'experts' as they may have more time to talk to you.

5. *Explore all the information about Parkinson's disease you can find* in journals, medical books, 'alternative' media, the Internet, from friends and associates.[21] Then sort that information into stuff you can readily understand, and stuff you need help with.

6. Then *sort the information* you understand into stuff that 'resonates' with you (ie. you feel comfortable with, and relate to what the writer is saying) and stuff to put aside for another time.

7. *Write down questions* about the information you need help with and seek answers from your GP, neurologist and any other health practitioner you are in contact with. If any practitioner can't or won't answer your questions, or tries to 'brush you off', perhaps they are not the right practitioner for you.[21]

8. *Sort out your priorities for treatment.* Do you want to find and treat the cause of your disorder (see 'What About Stress?'), or merely suppress the symptoms to help you

function for a while longer? If symptom suppression is what you want, then talk to your doctor about medication (see 'Medication'), and stop reading this book. If you want to work with the cause and try to regain better health, keep reading.

9. *Talk to your family and friends* about your feelings and your plans. Tell them how the diagnosis has affected you, and what you plan to do about regaining better health. Ask them to become part of your journey, to support you in your efforts and to be encouraging and observant.

10. *Start a journal.* Just ten minutes each week will help you keep track of your symptoms, what your health practitioners say, what sort of events make your symptoms worse and/or better. Write down your feelings too; this will really help along the way (see 'Your Journal – your second friend').[21]

11. Once you have gathered all the information you want, and have decided on the practitioners who will support the beginning of your journey to better health, *talk to each practitioner and ask them to communicate with each other*, and to be mindful of the benefits you receive from each type of therapy.

In my experience, **Western medicine and complementary medicine are entirely compatible for the treatment of Parkinson's disease. You DO NOT have to reject Western medicine if you choose complementary medicine, or vice versa.**

If you choose complementary medicine

If many neurologists are too gloomy and depressing about your prognosis, some complementary therapists are over-optimistic, and talk enthusiastically about 'curing' you.

Beware of these practitioners. There is no 'cure' for Parkinson's disease. You can, however, reverse the process of disease by working hard and gaining support from empathetic and experienced practitioners.

Find a naturopath or homeopath who:

1. *Is open-minded* about all the other therapies you wish to try, including Western medicine if that is your choice, and the practitioners you want to work with, and shows willingness to communicate with them.
2. *Shows a knowledge and understanding* of your disorder and how it affects you.
3. *Understands the very long-term nature* of this disorder, and is willing to work with you over a number of months and years, until you feel you can move on.
4. *Helps you take control of your life* and health, and supports you with kindness, respect and patience.

If any practitioner tells you they have a 'cure' for Parkinson's disease, or wants to get you involved in multi-level marketing ('network' marketing or 'pyramid' selling) on the basis of vague anecdotes of 'wonderful results', walk away; they are probably just going to cost you money with little or no return.

There are many complementary therapies and practitioners who will be helpful on your journey to better health. Search diligently, interview each practitioner and don't be embarrassed to say 'thanks, but no thanks' if it doesn't sit comfortably with you. YOU are the expert on your disease and body, and YOU are the best judge of who and what will help you the most.

8

Eating Well to Get Well

Recovering from any disease completely means improving the health of our whole person. In that sense, diet is important in recovering from neurological disorders. There has also been significant research into a diet to help control a particular form of Multiple Sclerosis, and this has shown a lot of promise.[22,23] However, I have not yet found a single dietary regime that has led to complete recovery from any neurological disorder.

That being said, it would be foolish indeed to ignore the great benefits gained from ingesting healthy, living food and the great improvements that this can bring in general health. I have included a few specific rules for particular conditions that have been shown to be beneficial, and suggestions for a dietary intake likely to enhance general health, and therefore improve our chances for recovery. You will also find lists of foods we know to be helpful and some we know to be harmful.

In considering any dietary changes we must remember that:

- People developing Parkinson's disease usually have poor absorption through the gut wall and, invariably, very poor cellular absorption. Therefore, we must improve absorption before we can expect to see full benefits from dietary changes. Some of this, especially at cellular level, is helped by the Aqua Hydration Formulas (described in a later

47

chapter), but we may need to work on our gut absorption to improve health.

- Each person has individual needs and these must be considered during long-term dietary changes.
- You may have particular difficulties in preparing food if you live alone. Your movements may be restricted, energy levels low, or balance uncertain, thus reducing your ability to prepare complex dietary requirements.
- Your carers may have particular dietary needs, restrictions or preparation abilities. If you rely on a carer for food preparation, please discuss any changes with them to gain their full understanding and cooperation.
- You may already be overwhelmed by your diagnosis, anticipated degeneration, frustration and fear at what is happening to you, and medication requirements, so dietary changes must be introduced gently and progressively to help you stick to them.
- Many of you may have lived on a particular diet for many years, and are in the habit of buying certain food, preparing it in particular ways, and may find it difficult to change your habits. But you can, given time and determination.
- There may be religious and/or cultural restrictions on ingesting certain foods.
- Some of you may be allergic or sensitive to some foods.

There is one rule that applies to everyone, especially those recovering from any form of serious illness:

ELIMINATE EXCITOTOXINS. These are chemicals added to foods and disguised under a variety of names – MSG, hydrolyzed vegetable protein, aspartame, 'natural flavouring', spices, yeast extract, textured protein, soy

protein extract and others. These chemicals are highly neurotoxic.

All processed foods contain one or more of these toxins. Even some of the 'good' food brands have added chemicals. READ THE LABELS.

'Diet' foods and drinks are particularly bad in this regard as they usually contain aspartame. DO NOT drink any 'diet' soft drinks, cordials, or purchase 'diet' jams, spreads, etc.

Buy a Food Additive Code Book, usually available from supermarkets, book stores and health food stores for a few dollars. Check the names and numbers of any additives you don't know with help from this book. You will be surprised at the poisons allowed into our food.

Dietary considerations for Parkinson's Disease

If you are diagnosed with Parkinson's disease and are taking levodopa (Kinson, Madopar or Sinemet) medication, there are dietary considerations for you to think about in order to gain the greatest possible benefit from your medication.

Medical practitioners place little emphasis on diet for the treatment of Parkinson's disease. Most literature makes no mention of diet at all except in relation to 'problems' such as constipation (high fibre) or nausea and vomiting (use an anti-emetic). However, low protein diets and protein redistribution diets have been investigated to see whether they potentiate the benefits of levodopa.

Levodopa, an amino acid, has to compete with other large neutral amino acids (LNAA) for transport in the small intestine and at the blood-brain barrier. The major competitors are phenylalanine, leucine, isoleucine, tryptophan, valine, methionine, histidine and tyrosine.

Croxson et al designed a study to discover the effect a diet of only 0.64 gram per kilogram of body weight of protein would have on Parkinson's symptoms while normal medication intake was maintained.[24] While this diet is low compared to Australian RDA (1 gram per kilogram of body weight),[25] it is not extreme and, therefore, sustainable over a long period. Some non-medical practitioners would argue that a lower protein diet is both sustainable and beneficial.

The Croxson study indicated that a low protein diet did improve motor function and reduced 'off' periods compared to a normal diet. This seemed entirely due to reduced competition of LNAA's with levodopa.[24]

Protein Redistribution Diets (PRD) limit protein intake during the day to 6–9 grams, but allow unlimited protein after 4pm.[26,27,28] The intention is to improve motor function during the day (assuming that this is when most activity is desired), while allowing the evening diet to make up any protein deficiencies.[26] The assumption is that the most common effects of LNAA competition with levodopa (akinesia, bradykinesia and freezing) will not be of such concern during the night time.[26] The PRD revolves around daytime intake of fruit, vegetable and fats, with minimal grain products. After 4pm, the emphasis is on protein, especially meat, fish, chicken and eggs.[26]

Several studies have identified benefits and problems with PRD. The major (and perhaps only) benefit is a significant increase in mobility and decrease in 'off' periods during daytime.[26,28] An important offset to these benefits was an increase in peak dose dyskinesia. In some cases this required a reduction of levodopa intake.[26,28]

The main disadvantages of the PRD are a very significant increase in nocturnal akinesia, and the fact that it only works in patients who suffer post-prandial (after eating) motor dysfunction. Those patients who are in stable symptom control with levodopa/carbidopa therapy gain no benefit from

PRD.[26,27,28] PRD patients have been observed for only 5 months or less, so there is little indication of long-term benefits or disadvantages. The most significant problem seems to be compliance, as patients tend to move off the diet after several weeks or less.[26,28]

Gimenez-Roldan and Mateo found that patients showing random 'on-off' periods and motor dysfunctions unrelated to meals were unlikely to benefit from PRD.[28]

Berry et al undertook a study comparing high protein and low protein diets with a diet of carbohydrates and protein in a 4:1 ratio. The study population was small (8 men) but the results indicate that this balanced diet may well be more efficacious than high or low protein diets because it is more nutritionally sound, and motor function either stays stable or marginally improves over the full 24 hours.[27]

While there is little to indicate particular advantages in severely reducing protein intake while taking levodopa supplementation, it is probably wise to experiment carefully with the timing of protein consumption, and observe the effect of the 'on/off' phenomena and dyskinesia.

General dietary suggestions

My own experience indicates that a 'naturopathic-nutritional' diet **high in omega 3 fatty acids**, and **very low in saturated fats, sugar and refined carbohydrates**, modified for your individual needs, is probably the most beneficial of all.

One of the best ways to start modifying your diet is to keep a **food diary** for two weeks. This is simply a notebook in which you write down absolutely everything that you eat and drink each day. Nobody has to see it except you, so you can be completely honest, noting those bits of chocolate you sneak in, two cakes instead of one, and the thick shake you had when no one was looking.

When you have all your notes for two weeks, compare your food intake with the list of 'Best Foods', 'Mediocre Foods' and 'Worst Foods' following. How much of your food comes from the 'Best Foods' list? 20%? 40%? We need to aim at consuming 70% of our diet from the 'Best Foods' list, and pad it out with 'Mediocre Foods'. We need to move away from 'Worst Foods' altogether.

If your diet is not actually toxic, it is better to make small changes over time rather than try to change everything at once. It is also important to involve your spouse/carer/family, especially if they are the primary food preparer, or if you are preparing meals for everyone.

If your spouse/carer is cooperative, it may be possible to construct a well balanced diet without too much trouble. But we can't take cooperation for granted. This is our journey and we must welcome our loved ones to the level of participation they can manage.

I consider a healthy diet to be based around fresh vegetables (raw or steamed), plus fresh fruit, nuts and seeds. Deep-sea fish three times a week, plus small amounts of lean meat (not processed).

Omega 3 fatty acids are most easily obtained from fish (especially cold water fish), flax seeds or flax seed oil and avocado. One or more of these foods should be eaten every day.

Dairy products may be replaced with goat or sheep milk and cheese if available, or Soy milk and yoghurt, Rice or Oat milk (in moderate quantities) if there is any hint of dairy sensitivity. While cows milk products contain a lot of calcium, most people find it very difficult to absorb as the milk protein is very large and may create inflammation around the gut, or change the permeability of our gut wall. It's not much good having lots of cows' calcium if we can't utilise it.

Calcium is more readily available from dark green vegetables (especially broccoli stalks), sardines, tuna, sesame seeds and a variety of other foods.

Eggs provide excellent protein and can be safely eaten several times each week. They are often maligned by people scared of cholesterol. However, we manufacture about 80% of our cholesterol endogenously and it is the ratio of HDLs to LDLs that is important. The cholesterol in fresh, free-range eggs is well utilised by most people. Eggs, as part of a sensible low-fat, high natural fibre diet, are good food.

Sugar, refined carbohydrates, food colouring and flavouring, and processed foods should be eliminated.

Diet drinks are particularly toxic as the aspartame sweetener is up to five times more active when combined with other drink ingredients. Aspartame, and the newer version known as Neotane, is one of the most neurotoxic chemicals known! Never consume it in any quantity.

Drink 1 to 2 litres (6 to 8 glasses) of clean, pure water daily (without fluoride or chloride if possible), plus diluted fruit juices, herbal teas and/or coffee substitutes.

Do you have to be super-strict?

How quickly do you want to restore your health? How much stress will it cause to be super-strict? In practice, I find it is easier to be 'good' with your diet if you select one day each week or fortnight to 'indulge' yourselves. This reduces the stress of being strict about your diet. I suggest you go out for brunch or lunch, and have that 'forbidden' cup of coffee or chocolate sweet. This makes it easier to stick to a healthy diet for the rest of the week.

However, those who establish excellent eating habits, focus on 'Best Foods' and who make few, if any, compromises, make better progress with their health.

Vegetarian, vegan, macrobiotic and similar diets can all enhance our path to health. However, for many people, the stress of planning, obtaining and preparing food for such diets outweighs their benefits. My philosophy is to work towards the healthiest diet possible consistent with the lowest possible stress for you and your family.

How to eat

The way we eat is almost as important as what we eat. Many of us have developed habits of rushing our meals so we can get back to 'more important things', or eating while doing something else – correcting papers, talking on the telephone, arranging dates, etc. This really confuses our body. We are busy producing chemicals to 'do the stuff' we are busy with, and trying to produce digestive chemicals at the same time. No wonder many of us suffer bloating, indigestion, reflux or poor digestion.

When your meal is prepared, sit quietly, either with your family or alone, and focus on the food, seeing the different colours and textures, feeling grateful for the nutrients it will provide for your health. Eat slowly, chewing each mouthful thoroughly (this is about half the digestive process, and allows your stomach to produce enough acid to process the food further, also reducing reflux). If you have company, talk about happy, peaceful topics; leave unpleasantness and argument for another time or your body will mistake eating for stress. If you are alone, you might want to play some soothing music, watch the birds outside your window, or just focus on the taste of the food you are eating.

When you have finished eating, sit quietly for a few moments, or go for a gentle walk in the garden or another pleasant place.

Reflux and bloating

Do you suffer from reflux, bloating or indigestion? Do you chew antacids or take a prescription medicine for reflux? The chances are you have TOO LITTLE acid in your stomach.

We need a very low pH in our stomach (less than pH 3) in order to process foods properly. If the pH is too high, food will not be broken down appropriately and may force its way back through the physiological oesophageal sphincter at the top of our stomach (ie. reflux), especially if our abdominal muscles and diaphragm are not well developed, or we sit slumped in our chair, or we rush around while eating or straight afterwards.

You don't need antacids! You need more acid! Here's a simple way to help. A few minutes before each meal (especially breakfast) squeeze the juice of half a lemon into a small glass of water at room temperature or slightly tepid. Drink this without haste, then eat normally.

If this doesn't resolve the problem, ask your naturopath/ herbalist for a small bottle of drops to assist your stomach performance. The herbs may include Chamomile, Poke Root (in very small quantities), Dandelion Root, or any of a number of other useful herbs. Six to fifteen drops in a little water before each meal will alleviate reflux, bloating and other digestive symptoms. You may wish to take some digestive enzymes (available from your health food store or supermarket) for a short time to help your digestive system return to efficiency.

Make sure you check with your doctor and/or naturopath to make sure there is no mechanical dysfunction or specific health condition causing your discomfort.

The following groupings of 'Best Food, Mediocre Food and Worst Food' have been prepared by Larisa Zoska, herbalist and medical ecologist from Canberra.

The best foods

The following foods will supply you with all the nutrients required so that your body can manufacture the proteins and glycoproteins necessary for its healing.

(Include as many of these as possible, at least 80%, as your staple and snack foods)

All vegetables:	(At least 70% of every meal recommended)
Best:	Fresh and steamed
OK:	Boiled, stir fried (in olive oil or water) or baked

Fruits that are high in fibre, and lower in sugar such as avocado, lemons, limes, tomatoes, cranberries, fresh figs, fresh apricots, kiwi fruit, pears, Granny Smith apples.

Fish:	(Especially deep sea fish). Canned fish is also good.
Best:	Steamed
OK:	Baked, fried (in a little extra virgin olive without batter)

Eggs – free range (organic if possible), boiled, poached, scrambled, fried in a little extra virgin olive oil.

Fresh whole nuts (but not peanuts) and seeds such as pumpkin seeds, sesame seeds, sunflower seeds etc.

Honey and **pure maple syrup**.

The following foods directly provide the complex protein and glycoproteins structures that heal.

Cold pressed seed and vegetable oils such as flax seed, olive oil, avocado oil etc.
NB. do not heat any oil except extra virgin olive oil, as heating changes the oil structure and may cause harm.

Herbs:
- as culinary herbs: (as many as palatable added to the vegetables and other food groups)
- as teas (such as dandelion, peppermint, rosehip etc.)
- as medicines – prescribed by a qualified herbalist or naturopath.

Mediocre foods

The following are foods that will not adversely affect your health, and will give you more energy value than nutritional value.

(These are fine as snack foods, and/or when the better quality foods are not available)

Fruits high in fructose (especially dried fruit). Avoid these if you have, or suspect you have, a fungal problem such as candida, diabetes or hypoglycaemia.

Lean young meat such as lamb or veal or game (organic is always better).

Soy milk and other soy products (in moderate quantities only), Rice milk or Oat milk.

Whole grain – especially oats, rye and barley, and possibly spelt (but not wheat).

Goat's cheese and milk, sheep's cheese.

The worst foods

The following foods give very little nutritional value, and have a mainly toxic value that counteracts any energy and nutritional value that they may have.

(Eliminate these from your diet as either staple meals or snacks, however once a week, for entertainment, a little of these may be OK – especially for the taste buds – check with your health practitioner.)

All dairy that comes from cows: (milk, cheese, cream, butter, yogurt).

Foods that have been processed in order to become a food such as margarine and processed meats such as bacon, ham, devon etc.

Food with additives (such as chemical preservatives, colours and flavours including artificial sweetener). *NB. never consume any artificial sweetener – it is neurotoxic.*

Coffee.

Most grains – especially wheat and refined cane sugar, and products made from grain such as breads, pasta, biscuits, etc.

Saturated fats (coconut milk, red meat, chicken).

Peanuts and cashews (can cause a reaction in certain people and cause bowel and digestive disruptions because of the moulds within the nuts that have a toxic effect once eaten).

Old or sick animals, or old and limp vegetables.

Supplements

Conservative therapists suggest that we can obtain all the vitamins, minerals and trace elements we require from a balanced diet. Clinical evidence and exhaustive scientific studies tend to refute this view. Our over-farmed soils have been neglected and abused for too many years to retain much nutrition to give to our foods. The overuse of fertilizers like super-phosphate, extensive use of herbicides and insecticides, plus broad-acre farming which allows top soil to be stripped by wind, have all conspired to deprive our plant foods of appropriate nutrients. Animals are intensively farmed, fed antibiotics and hormones to reduce disease and promote growth, and do not provide the nutrition we should be able to expect.

Therefore, I usually suggest some nutritional supplements. However, we must again temper our enthusiasm for high nutritional intake with recognition of your inadequate cellular absorption, limited financial resources and current pills-and-potions intake. Many people diagnosed with neurological disorders are already taking 10 to 20 pills each day for a variety of ailments and baulk at the idea of taking more. But some are useful and may, over time, help you to reduce your drug load.

Here are my suggestions for supplementation to assist recovery from neurological disorders. The list is by no means exhaustive or suitable for every individual. The supplements listed are aimed at enhancing your energy production or the function of brain cells, thus aiding recovery. Where other conditions, such as hypertension, arthritis, diabetes, ulcers or claudication exist, supplements may need to be modified to meet your more immediate needs, and you should talk to your chosen health practitioner about which supplement, and how much, is best for you.

The doses listed are for daily intake and should be modified to meet individual needs.

Vitamin C – *4000 mg, mixed ascorbates plus bioflavonoids, non-flavoured tablets or powder* – required for ground substance integrity, immune function, nutrient absorption and metabolism. It is a strong anti-oxidant and required for brain and nervous system function, also for retinal strength. Will help protect against hyperhomocysteinaemia (see the later chapter on MEDICATION).

Folic Acid – *500 mcg* – a must if you are taking any levodopa drug (see MEDICATION).

Co Enzyme Q10 – *100 mg* – strong anti-oxidant and enhances peripheral circulation, thus aiding brain repair, maintenance of even temperature in hands and feet, and may help reverse impotence.

Grape Seed Extract – *an amount equivalent to approximately 1 mg of procyanidins per kg of body weight if taken with synergists or 2 mg per kg of body weight if taken alone* – very powerful anti-oxidant. May be neuroprotective and assist in repair of brain cells. Studies have shown Grape Seed Extract to be more active and effective than the much lauded and very expensive Pycnogenol.

Vitamin B Complex – *high potency* – may assist in handling stress, maintenance of energy levels and metabolic function.

Vitamin E – *50 to 500 mg* – strong anti-oxidant that assists with peripheral circulation. Works synergistically with vitamin C. Use cautiously if there is any history of, or hint of heart disease.

Selenium – *5 mcg to 25 mcg* – good anti-oxidant, works synergistically with vitamin E. Deficient in most Western diets. May be toxic in very large amounts. Is often included in multivitamin supplements; read the label.

Zinc – *30 mg elemental Zinc* – deficient in most Western diets. Required for thousands of enzyme functions, cognitive function, prostate health, skin, etc, etc.

The supplements above are my preferences only and I **DO NOT** suggest you take them all. Talk to your chosen health practitioner about a level of supplementation that is practical financially and nutritionally.

Your Food Diary will show you and/or your health practitioner what nutritional deficiencies need to be overcome quickly, and this is where your supplement priority should be. However, as detailed in my later chapter on MEDICATION, vitamin C and Folic Acid (or a anti-homocysteine supplement) is a must if you are taking Kinson, Madopar, Sinemet or any other levodopa medication.

9

Household Chemicals

There are hundreds of thousands of man-made chemicals pumped into our environment every year. Some we know to be very dangerous, a few we know are relatively benign while, for most, we don't really know how they affect our bodies. Certainly there are many tests on rats and other animals before chemicals are released, and estimates of effects on humans are made from these tests. But rats are not humans, their response to toxicity is different, and there are no trials showing long-term effects on humans.

We learn about the dangers of environmental chemicals by tragedy. Insect sprays, fertilizers, pesticides, weed killers and many others released perhaps fifty years ago have been proven to be horribly dangerous to our health. It is only when many people die that our governments force companies to withdraw the offending substance.

We can't do much about that except lobby our governments tirelessly for greater safety and accountability. We can, however, clean up our house and personal environment.

Household chemicals have a profound effect on us because we are in contact with them day after day. Bleaches, detergents, cleaning products, deodorisers, shampoos, conditioners, furniture polish and many other common products all have toxic components.

Most robust people will not notice the effect household chemicals have on their body as they have the resilience to withstand the assault and, even if they feel a bit tired or 'off colour', will blame over-work, stress or 'a virus'. But, as people with Parkinson's disease, we are not robust. Our cells are much more fragile and vulnerable to attack by toxic chemicals. We may be one hundred times more sensitive to environmental chemicals than those in good health. Therefore, it makes sense to remove as many potentially harmful chemicals as possible from our immediate environment.

We have allowed large corporations and governments to impose thousands of poorly tested and potentially toxic chemicals on us without any protest. We have accepted the farce that producers of hair, dental and household products have our best interests at heart, and bought their products without reading or understanding the contents.

Producers of all the products we buy, safe or unsafe, exist only to generate profit for their shareholders. That is their legitimate reason for existence, and their legal right. I have no argument with that at all. Our mistake is that we believe advertising propaganda about their product, and their re-assurances of safety, without questioning their testing methods, thoroughness or motives.

Most products we buy for our personal or home use are tested only on animals (a very cruel and inhumane process), and/or on human tissue in laboratory conditions. Little, if any, testing is done on living humans in conditions of normal living. In contrast, homeopathic remedies, so often ridiculed by Western science, are tested on hundreds of human volunteers before being released onto the market.

Whenever you set out to purchase a personal care product or household product, here are a few suggestions to help you choose the safest:

1. Always read the label. Carry a small magnifying glass with you as much of the printing is very small. Always carry

your Food Additive Code Book as many of these chemicals are listed there.

2. If any of the contents are items that you can't pronounce, spell or understand, don't buy the product.

3. Some of the major contents to be avoided at all costs are *propylene glycol, sodium lauryl sulphate, sodium laureth sulphate (SLS), ammonium lauryl* and *laureth sulphate*, any *parabens*, any *propyl* no matter where it appears in a word, *methyl* whatever, *propanol, butylene glycol, butyl* anything, *aluminium* or *aluminum, sorbitol, peg*, and so on. There are between 14,000 and 20,000 toxic chemicals in our household and personal products alone that have the potential to cause or exacerbate serious illness.

4. Ammonium based products have the potential to exacerbate Parkinson's disease symptoms.

5. If the product has a strong perfume or aroma, don't buy it. Bleaches are particularly toxic, especially when we are fragile.

6. If the manufacturer claims that the product will 'clean without any effort on your part', don't buy it. It is relying on strong, potentially toxic chemicals to do the cleaning.

7. If the manufacturer spends thousands of dollars in main-media advertising (TV, daily newspapers, magazines and radio), examine the product very carefully. Manufacturers will only spend that sort of money on products that are capable of generating huge profits; that is, products that are cheap to produce but can be sold at high prices. Therefore, they are likely to contain cheap-to-produce synthetic components.

8. Don't use any personal care products (toothpaste, deodorant, etc.) that has strong perfume, or that is claimed will create an artificially perfect result quickly – that is, whiten

your teeth in fourteen days (bleach), make your hair shinier than ever (petrochemicals), keep you dry under-arm for twenty four hours while playing tennis in thirty seven degree heat.

Here are some suggestions for products and alternatives to help you live a comfortable and socially active life without poisoning yourself and your family.

Your house

- Dusting, glass cleaning and general cleaning can be done, generally, with microfibre cloths available from most supermarkets. Some of these products are promoted through multi-level marketing organisations but, in my experience, these are no more effective or durable that the much cheaper supermarket products.
- There are non-toxic cleaning products available from supermarkets, health food stores and specialist shops. Herbon make a wide range of cleaning and washing products that I have found effective and are sold in many Australian health food stores, while Orange Power and Citro Clean are available from supermarkets. Similar products are available in the USA, UK and Europe where they are widely advertised in the 'alternative' press, through health food stores, and promoted by naturo-paths. Don't be tempted by the claims of multi-level marketing products as there are always equivalents available for much less money.
- Other useful cleaning agents are hot water (you'd forgotten that one, hadn't you!), vinegar, eucalyptus oil (will clean almost any sticky substance off a hard surface), raw sea salt, pure soap, Bicarbonate of Soda, Borax (use sparingly) and lemon juice. Toothpaste (non fluoride, of

course) is very good for polishing metal surfaces – it was used to polish the windscreens of airplanes during WWII.

- Companies that manufacture herbal-based cleaning products also make washing up, dishwasher and laundry liquids without detergents as well as laundry powders. Commercial detergents can damage cell membranes and that's not good.

Your body

- Use pure soap for washing yourself. This can be obtained from health food stores and, sometimes, markets. Ask questions about how the soap is made, the contents and the perfumes used (if it is perfumed). Remember, when you are in warm water, your skin pores are open so you will absorb any chemicals more rapidly.
- Do not use any deodorant that contains aluminium (or aluminum). This is highly toxic and implicated in cancer, Alzheimer's and other neuro disorders. There are many non-toxic deodorants available if you need one. Many people have found they can go without deodorant by using pure soap for cleaning, drying themselves thoroughly and de-stressing their lives. However, if you are like me and sweat significantly on most days, a non-toxic deodorant is the go. Your body may take a week or two to adapt to the different action of your new product, so start using it a little more frequently. Be prepared to freshen up during the day if needs be – this is a nice time out to wind down a little. You will also find that, as you improve your diet and metabolic function, your body aroma will become more pleasant, even when you're sweating.
- Most commercial toothpastes contain fluoride (a commercial waste product recycled into your mouth for a profit) and either sodium lauryl (laureth) sulphate or

ammonium lauryl (laureth) sulphate. Avoid these. There are many toothpastes in supermarkets and health food stores around the world that are herbal based and free from nasty chemicals. Grants, Red Seal, Vicco, Weleda are just some of those products. Thorough, regular brushing with a soft brush, including your gums, will preserve your teeth as adequately as using the commercial, toxic toothpastes. Remember that your mouth is an easy entry for toxins too, and brushing makes it even easier to absorb chemicals.

- Make up and perfumes: avoid these as much as possible. I know you want to look your absolute best when attending special occasions, so look for certified organic make up products. Make sure that the seller and the product are certified as organic by an appropriate authority. Most of the time, you will be more beautiful if you go without. This will give your skin a chance to breathe freely and respond to gentle sunlight.

- Skin cleansers and moisturisers: Aloe Vera gel works well after washing in plain water or with pure soap. If you need a little help with skin healing, add some water miscible vitamin E liquid to the Aloe Vera gel, and work it gently into your skin each evening. Breathing exercises and laughter will improve your skin tone with no toxic effects at all.

- Hair shampoos and conditioners: avoid anything with sulphates or chemical names you can't spell or pronounce. When washing your hair, the pores of your head open, and chemicals are absorbed very readily. Your brain is just inside and that's what we're trying to heal. There are a number of excellent hair products available such as Herbon, Alchemy and Melrose (I have used all of these and found them good). There are many other brands, so read the labels carefully and experiment; talk to your local naturopaths and health food stores about products they have used and can obtain for you. As a bonus, when I changed from expensive commercial shampoos and conditioners (used because I thought my hair needed extra care as I got older) to herbal-based products, I found my hair became thicker and softer, and easier to manage.

- An alternative hair conditioner is apple cider vinegar diluted with water. Use about a tablespoon of vinegar per litre of water; rinse through your hair at the end of your shower and do not wash out. The aroma will fade as your hair dries soft and shiny.
- If you are in need of dental care, ask your naturopath or homeopath for remedies to help protect you from the toxic chemicals we can't avoid in dental surgeries. Ask your dentist to use acrylic fillings rather than amalgam. I know dentists say amalgam doesn't leak mercury, but let's not take chances; the other fillings work really well. Refuse fluoride cleaning – this is very toxic.

Your garden

- With a little thought and persistence, your plants will thrive in an organic garden. Read some books about growing plants organically and companion planting. If you need to kill weeds on pathways or when preparing areas of your garden, use boiling water (this knocks them out really quickly), then mulch heavily to prevent regrowth and enrich the soil.
- Never use any weed killers or pesticides – they'll do you a lot more harm than the pests.
- Soapy water is good for aphids, home-made garlic spray (pure soap, crushed garlic and water) will deter many

pests, and growing organically will attract birds and lady birds that will gobble up garden pests with relish.

- The best fertilizer is organic matter – compost, horse and chicken manure well composted and similar materials are far better, and kinder to us, than commercial fertilizers.

A gift for you

Your home and your body are where you live. They are, or should be, places of safety, kindness and love. You can create homes like this by using clean, natural, wholesome products. And, as a gift for you, you will enhance your health.

10

Rehydration –
Preparing the Environment

Water is absolutely vital for life. Maintenance of cell and plasma water volume, pH and electrolyte concentrations within narrow limits is essential for survival. Water continuously moves through cell membranes, from blood to lymph to plasma, and through the fascia,[29] transporting nutrients and extracting wastes. About 30% of our body weight is composed of intracellular fluid (fluid inside cells) which is mainly water. Another 20% of body weight is extracellular fluid (outside cells).

Homeostasis (the efficient balancing of our body's metabolic functions) requires that our water intake must equal its elimination via kidneys, liver, skin and respiration. This means that we must ingest a relatively large volume of hydrating fluids during each day in addition to the water we gain from food and cell metabolism. We need between 1.5 and 2 litres of water from all sources each day to maintain this balance. This includes fluids from fruit and vegetables, pure water, diluted juices and herbal teas. Most of us, during normal daily activity, need to drink around one to 1.5 litres of water, herbal tea and diluted juice to maintain optimum hydration

The science of hydration is in its infancy despite the fact that water is the single most important nutrient for our cells and biological systems generally.[30] The rate at which water moves into and out of cells establishes the efficiency of nutrient uptake, including oxygen, glucose, water-soluble nutrients and most fat-soluble nutrients.[30] Removal of waste products (cell 'detoxing') is also dependent on the rate at which water flows into and out of cells.[30] Any increase in water flow through our cells is likely, therefore, to improve our nutrient uptake, energy production and waste product disposal.[30]

Dieter Haussinger et al of the Heinrich Heine University in Dusseldorf, in a singular study on the effect of cell hydration on cell function, found that the level of cell hydration is the most important factor in determining whether cells display catabolism (tissue breakdown) or anabolism (rebuilding).[30] This is vital knowledge to those of us who display symptoms indicating cell destruction (eg. Parkinson's disease).

Our water intake depends, to a large extent, on our thirst reflex. Drinking occurs when the organum vascularis of the laminae terminalis (an area of the brain intimately connected to the hypothalamus) senses a reduced fraction of water in the cerebrospinal fluid.[30,31] Osmoreceptor cells in the hypothalamus detect these changes and initiate activity in neural circuits that give us a sensation of thirst, and stimulate behaviour seeking to redress our thirst.[30,31]

All too often, in Western society, we respond inappropriately to our thirst reflex. We may drink milk, tea, coffee or sugary soft drinks that may give a feeling of temporary reduction of thirst, but do not satisfy our body's need for hydration. We may mistake our thirst for hunger, and snack on something sugary or refined to give us an 'energy hit'.

When our thirst reflex is 'ignored', or we respond inappropriately for some time, our body 'learns' to ignore our thirst reflex. Thus we may no longer feel thirsty, and be blithely unaware that we are dehydrated. Sometimes, our body reacts by eliminating the feedback system that tells us when we have had enough to drink, so we become insatiably thirsty, but may continue to drink anything but water, thus exacerbating our dehydration.[30]

We also live in a very dehydrating society. Chemicals in our food, air pollution, eating and drinking habits, air conditioning and stress all rob our bodies of vital water. Even the water supplied in most Australian cities is modified with fluoride and chlorine that may, in fact, reduce our ability to utilise that water at cellular level and reduce our thirst sensation.

For our bodies to operate efficiently, we must both take in adequate quantities of water and be able to utilise this water effectively. This means that our bodies must be able to transport that water and other nutrients right into our cells to ensure the proper production of chemicals, disposal of waste products and transport of the chemicals produced to where they are needed.

By drinking too little water, we reduce the effectiveness of our physical defences. Our skin becomes dry, brittle and porous, and the patency of the mucus barrier in airways, lungs and gut is reduced, so allowing intruders (micro-organisms) to penetrate our first line of defence. Once inside our 'fortress', these intruders are faced by a very weakened immune system – weakened by the lack of water that slows transport of immune cells through fascia[29] and blood stream. Disease fighting cells are produced less efficiently and are slow to get to where they are needed because our lymph system and fascia transport systems have slowed down.

How much water?

We gain water through eating food with a high water content and consuming fluids. We lose water through perspiration, respiration, urine and faeces. We need to ingest and utilise sufficient water to replace the amount we lose each day.

If we eat a health-giving diet including a lot of fresh vegetables and fruit, and we are moderately active physically, we need to consume between one and two litres of water daily, depending on temperature and other environmental factors, to maintain homeostasis (a balanced metabolism).

As a rule of thumb, those still working and maintaining reasonable social activity should aim at consuming about 1.5 litres of pure water and/or very diluted fruit juice each day, while those who have left the workforce and are, perhaps, less active should aim at a minimum of one litre.

When temperatures are high, or your activity is promoting free perspiration and high respiration, water consumption needs to increase by around fifty percent.

How to enhance hydration

The **Aqua Hydration Formulas** began their development phase during the 1980's when Leonie Hibbert, a Melbourne based natural therapist, joined the growing number of health professionals who realised that dehydration was, probably, the single most important health problem of Western society, and set out on a journey of discovery to find better ways to redress this situation in individuals. Through research and consultation, Leonie developed a herbal/homeopathic protocol that assisted her clients to ingest and utilise water more efficiently. Originally, this consisted of a number of different and separate remedies to be taken twice daily – a kind of 'cocktail' of hydrating remedies.

In 1993, Dr. Jaroslav Boublik, a neuroendocrinologist, then a laboratory head at the prestigious Baker Medical Institute in Melbourne, consulted Leonie seeking help in preparation for running the Melbourne Marathon. He found that he kept 'hitting the wall' (ie. dehydrating badly) at about the 20 km mark and could not overcome this problem despite his best efforts. With Leonie's help, while maintaining his normal training programme, Jaroslav's hydration and performance improved so that he was able to complete the 1993 Melbourne Marathon in respectable time.[30]

Inspired by his performance and enhanced recovery rate, Jaroslav, Leonie and two other colleagues created Aqua-ConneXions, a research and development company with the intention of making the Aqua Hydration Formulas more convenient to use, efficient and commercially viable. With much research and development time, the Aqua Hydration Formulas finally became four remedies, specific for males and females, morning and evening.[32]

The **Aqua Hydration Formulas** (Aquas) have been developed to improve hydration by increasing both intake and uptake of water, thus improving metabolic function and elimination of wastes.

These formulas are designed to:

- reset the thirst reflex
- improve the bio-availability of water at cellular level
- improve hydration throughout the body
- work with emotional levels which may effect hydration.

I first 'discovered' the Aquas in 1997 while attending a lecture at my college (the Australian College of Natural Medicine), during which Jaroslav described the formulas and their intended function. At the time, I was still struggling with quite severe Parkinson's disease symptoms, and felt that I had reached a 'plateau' in my recovery pathway. I was much healthier than I had been at diagnosis in 1995, but still suffered incredible fatigue, severe tremor, poor speech, bad sleeping patterns, some incontinence, some postural hypotension and minor balance problems. I also 'felt crook' all the time (often described as 'general malaise').

Jaroslav's lecture inspired me to try these remedies – I believe I was the first person to use them for a Neurological Disorder – and I started the treatment with enthusiasm. There were some mistakes along the way as I was a 'guinea pig' for the use of these remedies for Parkinson's disease. However, with the support and understanding of Leonie and Jaroslav, I found a way to use the Aquas to enhance my recovery.

Theoretically, there are no contra-indications to using the Aqua formulas at the dosages suggested on the containers. In practice, it is not so simple and I have listed below some 'rules' and guidelines in prescribing the Aquas for those with Neurological Disorders that I have found to be useful in my practice.

The Aqua Hydration Formulas are at the heart of the RETURN TO STILLNESS recovery from Parkinson's disease programme. Rehydrating our bodies opens the way for the efficient production and utilisation of chemicals required for good health. However, it is important to be cautious in using the Aquas; people with neurological disorders are debilitated and sensitive, no matter how robust and confident we seem. The particular nature of neurological disorders brings great sensitivity to all medication, including herbs, homeopathics and flower essences – the components of the Aquas.

My experience in using the Aqua Hydration Formulas in the treatment of neurological disorders indicates that they bring the following benefits:

- increased utilisation of medications, bringing faster 'kick-in' and reduced 'off' times;

- increased energy levels;
- better sleep;
- improved bowel and bladder health;
- a greater sense of well being.

Benefits will vary with each individual, of course, and the full effect of hydration (when treating neurological disorders) may not be felt unless combined with Bowen Therapy, which I describe in a later chapter. However, if you are unable to attend a Bowen therapist, start the Aquas anyway and great benefits can accrue.

I must add a personal note here. I have no commercial interest in Wild Medicine, manufacturer and distributor of the Aqua Hydration Formulas, or production of the Aqua Hydration Formulas. I continue to promote the use of these remedies because they are the only way to achieve the results I see. However, if and when I find a better way, I will promote that just as eagerly.

The contents of the Aqua Hydration Formulas can be found in Appendix 2.

Using the Aquas

There are several ways of ascertaining the appropriate dose of Aquas for each person, and your health practitioner may help you to establish the right dose just for you. Whichever method you or your practitioner chooses, remember the one basic rule:

When there is any doubt, start at a very low dose.

1. **Vega Machines or similar** – these can be very useful in judging a person's sensitivity and need for any medication. It is relatively easy to test each individual to see where they should start with the Aquas, and how quickly

they should increase their dosage. However, the machine is only as good as the operator. If there is an indication for very high doses (7 or 9 drops, for instance), especially at the beginning, remember the basic rule. Testing should be for the requirement at CELL level, not organ level.

2. **Kinesiology/Muscle Testing** – another very useful and, potentially, very accurate way to ascertain the required dose. Again, remember the basic rule. I have experienced cases where muscle testing indicated huge doses (20 drops or more) which may well have ended recovery before it started. Fortunately, the clients concerned contacted me before starting the journey. Kinesiology is a wonderful modality, but is a tool to be used with discretion and love.

3. **Pendulums and similar** – again, wonderful, very useful modalities which can be very accurate. But, if in doubt, see the basic rule.

4. **Intuition/Psychometry** – this is my preferred method, but see the basic rule.

5. **Practitioner Prescribing** – prescribing by 'rule' is easy and safe. If this is the method you prefer, here is my suggested titration rate:

Week 1–2	1 drop morning and evening;
Week 3	2 drops morning, 2 drops evening;
Week 4 – and onwards	3 drops morning and evening;

Observe the effects of this dosage for some weeks before being tempted to raise it. Most people with Parkinson's disease stay at 4 drops or less for some time. If, after twelve weeks or so, there is still indication of chronic dehydration, it may be useful to increase the dose to 5 drops. It is very rare for anyone to need a higher dose. Indications of dehydration include chronic constipation with hard, dry stools; persistent or increasing nocturnal enuresis; thick, sticky mucus;

persistent edema; no reduction of 'kick-in' time for your standard medication. However, most signs of improvement at this stage are very subtle and it is best to be patient and cautious.

Wild Medicine, the manufacturer, suggests that the Aquas should be taken for five days each week with two days of rest because the formulas were designed to improve hydration in people who are basically well. This guideline, and the recommended dose of up to 7 drops morning and evening are reasonable for the general public. For people with Parkinson's disease, I have not found this useful until much later in the treatment. For at least two years, I ask my clients to take the Aquas every day. Because these remedies are primarily absorbed through the gut, rather than through our buccal membranes as with other homeopathic remedies, there seems to be no problem with 'proving' the remedies, a concern for some homeopaths who prescribe the Aquas.

On very rare occasions, the extra uptake of standard medication (eg. levodopa or other drugs), created by improved cellular absorption, has been so pronounced that adverse drug effects are noticed and I have asked clients to cease the Aquas for one week before recommencing on a lower dose. However, in most cases, reducing the dosage by one or two drops will alleviate any aggravation of drug-adverse effects that may be occurring.

'K' dilutions[33,34,35]

No matter how careful we are at selecting suitable dosage levels of the Aquas, some people will 'aggravate' after a few days to a few weeks. Signs of aggravation include exacerbation of your 'normal' symptoms, fatigue, irritability, the appearance of new or strange symptoms, or a feeling of being 'not quite right'.

Some people are extremely sensitive to homeopathic medicines at any time, and the onset of a neurological disorder seems to enhance that sensitivity. If you feel that you have reacted to homeopathic remedies in the past, or have difficulty in taking pharmaceutical medications, it may be wise to start the Aqua dosage at these 'K' dilutions.

Aggravation of symptoms when using the Aqua Hydration Formulas does not indicate any toxic or dangerous condition. These medicines are never toxic and never dangerous. The aggravation indicates that you are responding positively to the Aquas, but need only a tiny dose to achieve the desired result.

'K' dilutions are one useful way to gain this balance between benefit and aggravation. This method of remedy preparation was developed by a Russian homeopath, Semen Korsakov (1788-1853) who became interested in this modality some years before the great cholera epidemics in Europe (1830 and 1847).[35] Korsakov preferred his own method of preparation[33,34,35] over the precise dilution and succussion method perfected by Samuel Hahnemann, known as the Father of Homeopathy.[36,37]

Here's how to prepare 'K' dilutions:

K1

1. Put one drop of the appropriate Aqua into a glass of water.
2. Throw the water out but do not dry the glass.
3. Refill the glass with water and take a sip of this dilution each day at the appropriate time.

Does that seem too dilute to be any good? It works!

K2

1. Prepare a K1 dilution.

2. Throw away the water.
3. Refill the glass and sip as above.

Yes, this dilution works too.

To prepare **K3** and **K4** dilutions, repeat the steps above until you have thrown away the **number of glasses coinciding with the dilution number.**

The Aqua Hydration Formulas dosages used by my clients vary from as high as 5 drops morning and evening, to as low as K4 dilution, morning and evening three times per week. In each case, we have started with one drop morning and evening and observed the results carefully. If my client was comfortable, we moved the dose up by one drop each week until we reached five drops. If there was any hint of aggravation, we moved to K1 and observed for a week or two, and so on.

The Aquas will improve the uptake and utilisation of all other medications and supplements you are taking. Therefore, it may be necessary from time to time, to adjust the intake of these items. For details on this, see the chapter on MEDICATION.

The initial daily cost of the Aquas is very small (less than 60 cents per day in Australia), very little for the benefits gained. They should be treated respectfully as any other homeopathic medicine – stored away from direct sun, heat and sources of electro-magnetic radiation.

Some health food stores and pharmacies carry the Aqua Hydration Formulas as retail lines. Many naturopathic practitioners have realised the benefits of the Aquas for numerous health conditions and maintenance of robust health, and stock them in their practice. However, if you have any difficulty in obtaining supplies of Aqua Hydration Formulas, contact the manufacturer, Wild Medicine Pty

Ltd, or Return To Stillness (see USEFUL WEBSITES AND OTHER RESOURCES).

The Aquas are powerful, energetic medicine, which greatly enhance our ability to reverse the symptoms of Parkinson's disease.

What sort of water?

Water is one of the recent marketing targets, and we are badgered by advertising claiming miraculous properties for all sorts of manufactured water. There's water with oxygen, water with minerals, miracle water, magic water, you-bewt-we're-going-to-charge-you-heaps-for-this water, and alkaline water to name a few.

Don't get stressed out about the need to buy expensive water with fancy advertising, it's NOT necessary. The water we need is really simple to visualise. Imagine a mountain stream bubbling over rocks as it flows through pristine rain forest with sun glinting off the ripples; or a spring bubbling up between rocks of a grassy mountainside. That's perfect water for our needs, but hard to obtain for most of us. We can get fairly close though.

I suggest you try to avoid fluoridated water as this chemical is very dehydrating and quite toxic, lacking any real proven health benefits. Chlorine may also be dehydrating and/or toxic. However there are three simple ways to obtain good, clean water:

- Buy a good quality filter and attach to your tap, or install it online. Costs vary very significantly so shop around. You want a filter that will remove 95% or more of the fluoride and chlorine. Some bench top filter jugs can do this well too. Change the filter very regularly.
- Buy spring water from the supermarket. Yes, much is in

plastic that may offset the benefits very slightly, but it is much better than straight tap water in cities that choose to add fluoride to their water supply. I buy 15 litre containers of spring water for around A$6.50 (in 2005), and that lasts me a week, including water for my clients.

- Install a rainwater tank with a small filter to eliminate any pollutants. There are tanks available today that reject the first 'flush' of water so that your roof is cleaned for a few minutes before the water starts flowing into your storage tank. This combined with a simple filter will provide very good water for drinking.

- *By the way, don't be tempted to boil fluoridated water thinking this will remove the chemical. Fluoride is heavier than steam, so stays in the water while it's being boiled, and is, in fact, in higher concentration after the process.*

- Alkaline water just doesn't make sense. Remember, we need a lot of acid in our stomach to process food properly. You may also remember that one of the effects of long-term stress is alkalosis (a pH that is too high), and this can be a very challenging condition. If we drink alkaline water, we reduce the available acid in our stomach, and increase the possibility of developing alkalosis. So don't waste your money.

11

Relaxation, Contemplation, Meditation and Spirituality

People with Parkinson's disease share two very basic emotions – fear and frustration. We are frustrated that we can no longer do all the things we used to do, or do them as well as we used to, and we are afraid that we will continue to get worse and be able to do less and less. These feelings are present no matter what symptoms are manifesting.

Often other emotions seem to loom large as well. Diagnosis may bring out forgotten memories, or we may relate the progress of the disorder to events in the past, rightly or wrongly. Regrets or sadness may well up unexpectedly because diagnosis changes our life so dramatically.

There are a number of ways to deal with our emotions. Some are, in my opinion, better than others.

Many conservative therapists will either ignore the emotional state of their patient, concentrating solely on the physical, or prescribe anti-depressants. The former exacerbates our frustration because we really do want to talk about it and find strategies to overcome it; the latter merely covers up an emotional situation that can be used to bring about a healthy life change. Most anti-depressants also have the potential to exacerbate some symptoms of Parkinson's disease,[1] thus increasing the underlying fear and frustration.

Other therapists see that there are emotional issues to be dealt with, and refer their patient to a psychiatrist.

Sometimes this is very successful, especially if the psychiatrist is empathetic and has a good understanding of the frustration and fear associated with a chronic, degenerative, ostensibly incurable disorder. However, many psychiatrists rely heavily on medication to achieve desired results and, again, I must state that I feel this type of therapy is counterproductive.

Emotional counsellors of many modalities can be of enormous help as outlined in the section on Depression. People who have or are working with me have found help from psychologists, trained counsellors, pranic healers, hypnotherapists, ministers of religion experienced in counselling, flower essence counsellors, and many others.

There are, however, ways to help ourselves work through, and overcome, these emotional onslaughts. A variety of relaxation techniques, meditation and contemplation can bring an awareness of the positive aspects of our lives and help us find a 'peaceful space'. It is important to note that *all those who have fully recovered from any neurological disorder have spent a great deal of time and dedication in meditation and personal/spiritual development of some sort. Those who recover from other ostensibly terminal diseases display similar dedication to the development of peace and an awareness of their own strength and beauty.*

Meditation was considered weird, whacky and way out by conservative therapists for many years. It is, after all, an ancient art, and most Western scientists and doctors felt it had no place in modern medicine.

Studies over the past few years, however, have changed that perception dramatically. We now know that meditation, practiced daily over time, can help us maintain or regain health.[21,38,39,40] Controlled trials, open surveys, medical examinations and electroencephalograph (EEG) studies are all showing positive health benefits for those who meditate regularly.[21,38,39,40]

Dr Jon Kabat-Zinn, Associate Professor of Medicine in the Division of Preventive and Behavioural Medicine at the University of Massachusetts Medical School, conducts eight-week courses called the Stress Reduction and Relaxation Programme in the University of Massachusetts Medical Centre.[38] Those completing the eight-week programme, and practicing meditation at home daily, find that their illness symptoms reduce by an average of 37 percent without any change to treatment except practicing meditation.[38] The Stress Reduction and Relaxation Programme does not focus on any person's condition or specific symptoms; participants learn to meditate in a certain way, and practice that daily.

A controlled pain study by Dr Kabat-Zinn in this programme followed two groups of people suffering chronic pain and being managed in the hospital's pain clinic using standard Western pain control medication. Twenty-one people using only Western medication were followed for ten weeks, while another twenty-one people participated in the Stress Reduction and Relaxation Programme and were also followed for ten weeks. It was found that the meditators gained a 37 percent reduction in pain while the non-meditators showed no improvement. There were similar significant benefits in body image and psychological stress for those meditating.[38]

Long-term studies have shown that meditation can lower levels of stress hormones such as adrenaline (one of the chemicals implicated in the onset of Parkinson's disease) and this can have beneficial effects on blood pressure and cholesterol levels.[39] EEG studies show that meditators show improved blood circulation, lowered levels of lactic acid (leading to reduced pain and anxiety), reduced heart rate and enhanced immune systems.[39]

Dr Herbert Benson MD of Harvard has noted that those who meditate or 'go into a quiet state' have fewer medical symptoms.[39] Dr Jill Marjama-Lyons, a neurologist from Jacksonville, Florida, says that 'recent studies in psychoneuro-immunology show that the mind can communicate with the nervous, immune, and endocrine systems.'[21] . . . 'mind-body techniques are particularly useful in the stress-reduction areas, helping to reduce blood pressure, pain, headaches, asthma, and other illness with a strong stress component.'[21]

In the previous section 'WHAT ABOUT STRESS?' I explain the probable link between unresolved traumatic stress and the development of Parkinson's disease. It makes a lot of sense, therefore, to enthusiastically participate in any activity that is known to reduce or ameliorate the bad effects of stress, while being non-toxic, cheap, pleasant and allowing you to be in control. You have much to gain by meditating, and nothing to lose.

Meditation comes in many forms and you can choose the one that suits you best. The suggestions below are just a sample of what is available for you, and may help you find your way to the type of meditation/relaxation technique that gives you the most benefit.

Regular walks in peaceful places

I will talk about the benefits of regular exercise, including walking, in a following chapter. Finding a place to walk that is peaceful and welcoming – eg. parks, by the sea, along a quiet street where there are beautiful gardens, beside a river – can help calm our tumultuous emotions. The exercise itself has a calming effect while the surroundings enhance this and encourage us to walk a little longer.

If you are not able to walk far, or cannot find a quiet place, try these other techniques.

Breath work

There are a number of breath work techniques that assist in bringing calmness and strength to our emotions and bodies.

It is not within the scope of this book to direct you to every breath work venue, but there are many advertised on the World Wide Web, plus many more in Alternative/ Complementary/New Age publications.

You may find this simple process useful: *Spend five minutes, two or three times daily, focusing your eyes on a beautiful scene or picture, then breathing deeply and slowly. Breathe in through your nose; feel as if you are filling your abdominal cavity with air by pushing your diaphragm out and down. Hold your breath momentarily, then exhale slowly through your mouth. Pause for a second, then repeat the process. As you do this over and over, your thoughts will become calmer, and your body will feel more relaxed. Remember to allow your shoulders to 'drop' and relax while you are breathing.*

Contemplation

For those who are relatively immobile and/or not practiced in the art of meditation, contemplation is a very calming and healing practice. Choose your favourite peaceful music and find a quiet place in your home in which to play it. Then you can sit either just listening with your eyes closed and allowing the music to drift through you, or you may like to look at beautiful pictures of landscapes, flowers or trees. If you are lucky enough to have a beautiful view from your window, then this is a bonus. Steady, deep breathing while listening (see 'Breath work' above) will enhance the benefits.

Meditation

There are many forms of meditation, and all are valid, health-giving techniques. I suggest that you find a teacher or group to suit your physical and philosophical needs. In my experience, it is more important to feel at home in a meditation group than participate in any particular form of meditation, no matter how powerful or focused a specific technique may be.

Some of the many types of meditation available are:

Guided meditation This is particularly good for those unused to meditation, or who come from conservative backgrounds. The leader guides class members on a 'journey' in their minds, creating word pictures that allow each member to interpret them in their own way, yet enjoy the peaceful energy created by the group. There are many CD's and tapes available to enable you to participate in Guided Meditation at home.

Unguided meditation with a leader For those who feel comfortable meditating by themselves, but enjoy being with a like-minded group, and benefit from feedback. The leader makes sure that everyone is getting the most from their meditation, supports those needing reassurance, and can lead discussion on individual meditations if the group desires this.

Unguided meditation without a leader Great for people who enjoy meditating at home, but like to join with others on a regular basis for the extra 'energy' generated by like-minded people.

Spiritual development meditation An advanced form of meditation conducted by an experienced spiritual leader who is able to teach the group about developing their individual strengths, and interpret sensations or visions that may occur during individual meditation.

Individual meditation Important for anyone seeking to gain benefit from any form of meditation. Individual meditation on a daily basis (at least) brings peace and strength from our own resources which may lie hidden until we undertake this type of discipline.

Prayer Prayer is a conversation with God, however we may interpret that concept. Each person will pray in their own way and gain the benefits they expect. Prayer can be as powerful as meditation in bringing healing change if that is what we want and expect.

Those from mainstream religions will pray to the God they know by name, others will pray to the Universe, Universal Love, the Great Spirit, or to their own Higher Being. I believe that there is no difference. Most accept the presence of a great creative force and understand that we are part of that force in some way. Praying to our accepted Godhead brings great benefit in focusing our energies on the road to health. However, it is important to pray with responsibility. God cannot help us if we ignore all the wonderful resources placed around us.

There are many ways for people with Parkinson's disease to help themselves. I encourage you to explore anything that intrigues or interests you.

12

Laughter – Internal Jogging that Exercises the Body[41]

We all know that laughing makes us feel good. We enjoy chuckling, giggling, laughing out loud, a good belly laugh. But we don't always realise why we feel good.

Scientists studying the physiology of laughter have found that many of the chemical changes that happen during laughter are the same as those that occur during exercise.[21,41] Endorphins (our natural painkillers) and many neurotransmitters are boosted during laughter, while stress hormones like cortisol and adrenaline are suppressed.[21,41,42]

There's even better news. Laughter improves our immune system. Cells that produce antibodies, T-cells and natural killer cells increase in number[21,41,42] while gamma interferon and immunoglobulin A are preserved or increased in production.[41,42]

So laughter not only makes us feel good, it IS good for us. Our pain levels may reduce and our immune protection increase if we laugh for just a few minutes each day.[41,42]

Okay, you're feeling pretty down about having Parkinson's disease, you're struggling to do many of the things you used find enjoyable, and you just don't see that there's much to laugh about. Don't worry about it, PRETEND to laugh; even faking a laugh will bring about the physiological changes that are good for us.[41] Even better, watching humorous movies, hearing jokes or reading funny books without laughing will still bring positive changes.[21,41]

Choosing to watch, hear or read the humour we like also boosts our sense of control, an important part of feeling healthier.[41,42] People recovering from surgery in a Florida hospital who were allowed to watch their favourite funny movies needed less painkillers that those who watched no humour or who had to watch what they were told.[41]

Laughter can boost our immune system, reduce pain, exercise our body and make us feel good. There are no toxic side effects and laughter costs nothing! What's the catch? We don't do it enough!

Children playing around in a safe environment laugh between 300 and 400 times each day.[21,41] As adults, we laugh, perhaps, fifteen to seventeen times daily.[21,41] What a reduction in self-help that is! Just by laughing, or PRETENDING to laugh thirty times each day, we can double all the benefits. Thirty seconds per pretend laugh equals only fifteen minutes per day for all those benefits. And we gain a sense of control, which further boosts our feeling of well-being.

This all sounds like a hard sell on television, doesn't it; 'and here are the steak knives'. Laughter may help us look better. Susan Welch, a certified Laughter Therapist and director of Authentic Happiness Australia, says that 'fifteen minutes of laughter stimulates the blood supply to the face'; and 'a good laugh oxygenates the body, nourishing the skin and reducing that tired look.'[43]

Now you're convinced that laughter is among the best and cheapest medicine you can get, what are you going to do about it? Here are some suggestions:

- Make a 'comedy evening' each week with your family, hire funny videos or DVD's, watch them together with a little of your favourite 'treat' food. Laugh out loud at the funny bits, even if you don't feel like it.
- Buy a giant joke book, and read at least two pages every day. Go back over your favourite jokes twice per week. Laugh out loud, even when people are watching.
- Get together with family or friends and play 'remember when' – *remember when Dad fell in the fish pond* (laugh); *remember when I was learning to ride a horse and I got on one side and fell off the other* (laugh); *remember when Mum accidentally sprayed under her arm with fly spray instead of deodorant* (laugh).
- Meet with three or four friends each week and tell jokes, even the old ones that you have heard over and over for years. Laugh at every joke, even if you don't think it's funny on the day. If the joke is told badly, laugh because it was told so badly (even if you told it).
- Save some of the thousands of funny jokes, pictures and movies that circulate in cyberspace in a special 'laugh' folder. Log into this folder every day and read or watch at least five items in there.
- Make faces at yourself in a mirror for three minutes every day.
- Join a 'laughter workshop'. Sounds like hard work, I know, but it is actually hilarious fun to be with a group of people who just want to laugh and be silly.
- If you can't find a 'laughter workshop' convenient to you, get a group of friends together and hire someone to run it for you – check the internet for lots of contacts to help you find a therapist; or ask around, many people who work for children's charities know the value of laughter and can help you.

- Think about children laughing. Happy and healthy kids laugh when they see a butterfly flutter around a flower, when Teddy falls off the couch, when the dog barks at the cat and the cat jumps, when they drop food on the table cloth, when Granny farts. Pretend to be a kid again and laugh at everything.

One last benefit of laughter is that it can, and will, improve your relationships. You can't be angry or bitter at someone if you laugh together. If you laugh a lot, and feel childlike and joyful, you don't even want to feel sad or angry or negative or left-out or any of those other feelings that fracture relationships. You just want to be with that person who laughs when you do and makes you want to laugh more. Victor Borge, that king of comedy in music, says 'Laughter is the closest distance between two people.'[44]

Go on, laugh, it can only make you well.

Happiness

Happiness is two kinds of ice cream, finding your wardrobe
    key, telling the time
Happiness is learning to whistle, tying your shoe again
Happiness is clapping your hands in a game
And happiness is walking hand in hand

Happiness is two different crayons, finding a secret, climb-
    ing the stairs
Happiness is finding a dollar, catching a butterfly, then set-
    ting it free
Happiness is being alone every now and then
And happiness is coming home again

Happiness is morning and evening, daytime and night time too,
For happiness is anyone, and anything at all that's loved by
    you.

Adapted from a poem written by an unknown author

13

Exercise

Our bodies need activity (exercise) to function efficiently. Our blood circulation, lymph drainage, elimination systems and even some chemical production depend on, or are helped by regular exercise.

If we use our muscles regularly, they will remain as strong and flexible as our overall health will allow. If we neglect them, and sit around doing nothing all day, they will grow weaker and weaker until we have very little strength left. Our joints need movement too. Moving joints remain more flexible for longer than joints that are still.

Parkinson's disease often restricts our ability to participate in the activities we are used to, so the temptation is to do very little, or nothing. But, even if our level or type of activity is restricted, we can still be active and enjoy it.

Perhaps our balance is a bit 'wonky'. Perhaps we've lost some of our muscle strength or coordination. Perhaps we feel we can no longer support our teammates as before. This is disappointing, but we can still take part in healthy, enjoyable exercise, no matter how our body is manifesting symptoms of a neurological disorder.

The **advantages** of regular exercise that is as energetic as our body will allow are:

- assimilation, utilisation and elimination of food are improved
- low density lipoproteins ('bad' cholesterol) are reduced

and high density lipoproteins ('good' cholesterol) are increased

- lymph circulation is improved, helping avoid fluid retention and assisting immune function
- other immune cells circulate more rapidly, so are more effective
- blood circulation is improved, helping maintain a good blood pressure and protecting blood vessels
- your heart and lungs become stronger and more effective
- bone density is improved
- muscle tone is increased
- your joints remain flexible and pain free for longer
- you will feel better about yourself and cope better with stress

The **disadvantages** of sensible regular exercise are: **NONE**

If you have not exercised for a long time, or if you have other disorders such as heart disease, lung disease or arthritis, discuss your exercise plans with your health practitioner. Exercise will still be good for you, but may need to be tailored especially for your circumstances.

Types of exercise

Probably the best kinds of general exercise are walking, swimming and dancing. Within those three classifications there are a large number of variations.

WALKING – walking by the sea or through parks; power walking around the suburbs; walking the dog; walking with your family; walking with a friend.

SWIMMING – swimming laps in a pool; swimming in the sea; playing water polo; playing volley ball in a swimming pool; swimming with your family.

DANCING – ballroom dancing; modern dancing; Latin dancing; rock and roll; old time dancing; line dancing.

Social exercise such as tennis, golf and cricket are all wonderful variations on this theme.

Yoga and Pilates classes are wonderful ways to help your strength and balance while exercising. Talk to your instructor about adapting the exercises to suit your level of mobility and strength.

Many people enjoy working in a gymnasium doing either weight work or aerobic exercises, or a combination of the two. Talk to your instructor about what Parkinson's disease means to you and how it affects your body. Make sure they understand that you need to work slowly and progressively as you move toward greater wellness. If you feel that the instructor doesn't quite understand, you may want to ask your health practitioner to write a letter, or speak to them. When you help yourself in this way, you may be helping others who approach the same instructor with particular challenges.

If your mobility and strength do not allow you to participate in such energetic exercise, there are other activities that can help you, no matter what your physical condition may be.

For those who have limited mobility

Cross-crawling, limb movements and flexibility movements, with or without help, will be of benefit. Start with the stretches shown below to the level of your ability. As you grow stronger and more flexible, you will be able to increase the number of repetitions of each exercise and, perhaps, move on to some more advanced activities.

For those who are a bit mobile:

An exercise bike or treadmill can be useful. Do short periods of exercise (say 5 to 10 minutes) twice daily. Create a 'walking circuit' around your house and traverse that a set number of times each day, increasing by one or two circuits each week. You might decide to walk from your lounge room into the hall, down the passage, into the kitchen and back into the lounge five times at first. Then increase to six times next week and so on.

The Best Time to Exercise is before meals. Do your most energetic activities before you eat, then rest for at least half an hour after your meal.

Everyone can do some exercise, even if you are confined to bed. It will make you feel better, and will help improve your health. So, go on, get energetic!

Stretching exercises for those with limited mobility

We introduce all participants, on a voluntary basis, at our Neuro Recovery Pathways programmes at the Quest For Life Centre to these exercises shown below. Everyone who persists each morning (just four mornings), improves significantly in flexibility, balance and strength, while often reducing pain and feeling triumphant at their achievement.

Starting the day

While still in bed, lie on your back, kick your covers off and do some cross-crawling.

1. Lift your left leg, with your knee bending, as

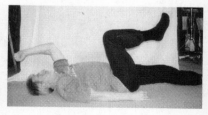

high as you can (as if crawling) while lifting your right arm over your head.

2. Lower these limbs and repeat using your right leg and left arm.

3. This exercise is like imitating a beetle on its back trying to crawl.

4. Do this ten to twenty times each morning to gain flexibility and encourage circulation before getting out of bed.

When you're ready, start some serious stretches.

Begin with breathing

1. Breathe in through your nose; feel as if you are filling your abdominal cavity with air by pushing your diaphragm out and down.

2. Put your hands on the upper part of your abdomen and feel it push out against your hands.

3. Hold your breath momentarily, then exhale slowly through your mouth.

4. Pause for a second, then repeat the process.

5. As you do this over and over, your thoughts will become calmer, and your body will feel more relaxed. Remember to allow your shoulders to 'drop' and relax while you are breathing.

Become a rag doll

1. Let your hands and arms hang loose beside you and feel your shoulders drop and relax.

2. Shake your hands, arms and shoulders so you flop around like a rag doll.

3. If you are able to stand securely, let your body flop around too. Feel loose and relaxed all over.

Back stretch

1. Sit as far forward in your chair as you can while feeling safe and secure. Keep your feet flat on the floor about your shoulder width apart with a small stool (or pile of books) between your feet.

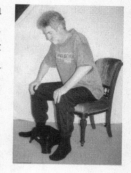

2. Put one hand on each knee and take your weight on your hands and arms.

3. Lean forward, keeping your weight on hands and arms.

4. Move your left hand from your knee to the stool, keeping your weight on your right arm, bending only as far as needed to reach the stool.

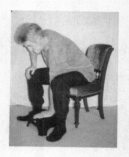

5. Take all your weight on your left arm (on the stool), then move your right hand from your knee to the stool.

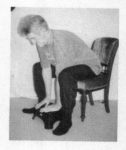

6. Take your weight evenly on both arms. Feel the muscles in your back stretch gently.

7. Move your left hand back to your knee, keeping your weight on your right arm.

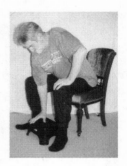

8. Transfer your weight to your left hand (on your knee) and move your right hand back to your knee.

9. Repeat four or five times, remembering to take all your weight on your arms. This will stretch your back muscles without causing any damage or pain to your back. You can adjust the height on the stool/books to suit your level of flexibility.

Mid back twist

This exercise frees up the muscles of your middle back, and will enhance flexibility of movement. You will need to be seated on a chair with a solid back to be safe.

1. Sit facing back on your chair with your left leg pressed against the back.

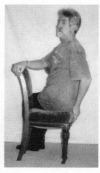

2. Keep your back straight, but relaxed, and twist to your left, grasping the back of the chair with your right hand.

3. Grasp the base of the chair with your left hand, then gently pull yourself towards the left using both hands for movement and balance.

4. Hold for one long breath, relax, then do it again.

5. Repeat this exercise on the right side.

6. Do not twist beyond your comfortable balance or if you feel pain.

Hamstring stretch and quad lift

This is a basic exercise to stretch your hamstring muscles and develop strength in your upper legs while seated. At the end of this section, you will find alternative ways of doing these exercises.

1. Sit squarely on your chair with your bottom pressed to the back. Hold onto the sides or arms of the chair for balance if you need to.

2. Extend one leg onto a stool or pile of books in front of you.

   Keep your leg straight but your foot relaxed. Keep your other foot squarely on the floor for balance.

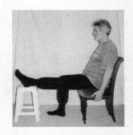

3. Pull back with the toes of your elevated foot to stretch your hamstring muscles. Do this three or four times.

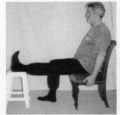

4. With your toes pulled back, lift your leg from the stool to strengthen the muscles of your upper leg (Quads). Do this one to four times depending on your ability. Don't worry if you can only lift your leg a couple of centimetres any movement helps.

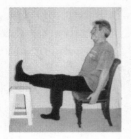

Sciatic stretch

1. You may need support to do this exercise, or assistance in achieving the correct position.

2. Sit diagonally on your chair so that one buttock 'falls' off the front edge. This is safer if your chair has arms to give stability.

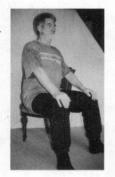

3. Lift the 'outside' leg and place your ankle across your 'inside' knee.

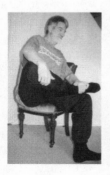

4. Keep your back straight while leaning forward until you feel your hamstring muscle and sciatic nerve stretching.

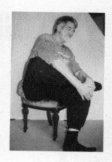

5. Hold for ten seconds, then sit back.

6. Repeat this three or four times before changing position to stretch the other leg.

7. This is a very useful exercise if you have pain in the buttock/sciatic area, or hamstring cramping.

Upper and mid back stretches

Here are two versions of an exercise to stretch all the muscles of your upper and mid back

Version one

1. Sit upright on your chair, looking straight ahead.

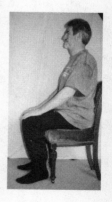

2. Allow your head (only your head) to droop forward towards your chest.

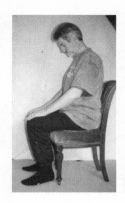

3. Grasp the top of your head with your hands and hold it in position.

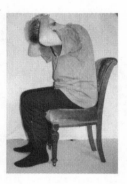

4. Push your back and hips backward to stretch the muscles in your mid back.
5. Repeat this three or four times. Stretch only to the limit of your comfortable stretch.

Version two
1. Sit upright in your chair.

2. Reach forward and grasp your knees with your hands, allowing your head to droop forward at the same time.

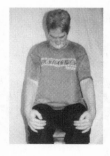

3. Pull your shoulders forward with your hands while keeping your back straight.

4. Roll your hips backward to stretch your mid back muscles.

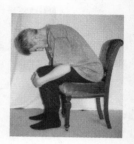

5. Repeat three or four times.

Reverse mid back stretch

1. Sit with your chair facing a wall, far enough away to let you lean forward, but close enough to be safe. Put your feet flat on the floor as far apart as you comfortably can.

2. Reach up as high as you can with your hands a shoulder width apart, and rest them firmly on the wall, looking at a point between your hands.

3. Pull down against your hands with your back muscles and feel the stretch.

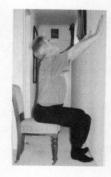

4. Return to the original position, then arch your back in towards the wall.

5. Repeat three or four times.

Head and neck stretch

1. Sit straight in your chair and hold the side or arm of the chair with your left hand.

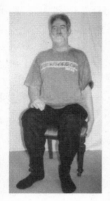

2. Gently move your head towards your right shoulder – do not move your shoulder.

3. Raise your right hand and hold your head in position. Do not pull the head at this point.

4. Push your head to the left against the pressure of your hand. Breathe in and out slowly, then release pressure.

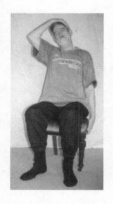

5. Gently pull your head to the right with your hand.

6. Repeat 3 and 4 slowly and gently until you feel you have moved your head as far as you comfortably can on that day.

7. Now hold the chair with your right hand and repeat this process to stretch your head to the left side.

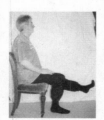

Hand and foot loosener

1. Sit with one foot flat on the floor and your other foot stretched in front of you.

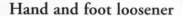

106

2. Rotate your extended foot outward four times, then inward four times. Rotate to the full extent of your flexibility.

3. Now put that foot flat on the floor, extend your other foot and rotate.

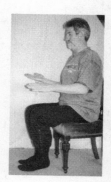

4. Hold your hands in front of you with your elbows bent at right-angles and close to your sides.

5. Rotate your hands outwards four times and inwards four times.

Alternative hamstring and quad stretches

These stretches are useful alternatives if you are certain of your balance and/or can rise from kneeling without trouble.

Hamstrings

1. Stand behind your chair, holding to the back as shown, with your feet about shoulder width apart. Your hands should rest easily on the chair back without having to reach too far forward. Make sure your chair is secure and will not tip backwards.

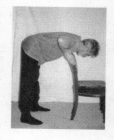

2. Take your weight on your arms, and lean forward with your legs straight. Feel the hamstring muscles stretch. Lean forward until your chest touches the back of your chair if this is possible.

3. The amount of stretch can be increased by moving your bottom back a little without moving your feet.

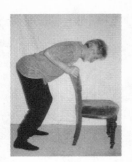

4. To rise from this position, bend your knees first, then use your legs and arms to push you upright.

Quads – kneeling

1. Kneel in front of your chair with your weight mostly on your arms.

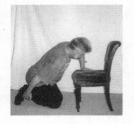

2. Transfer your weight to your left arm, then reach down by bending to the right, and pick up your right ankle.

3. Using your left arm to do the work, slowly push yourself up stretching your right quad muscle as you do.

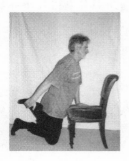

4. Repeat on the left side.

5. When finished, use your arms to help you rise to your feet without straining your back.

Quads – standing

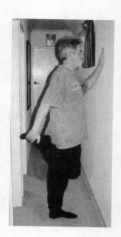

1. Stand facing a wall so that you are fully supported in an upright position.

2. Take your weight on your left arm, then reach down with your right hand while lifting your right leg, and grasp your ankle.

3. Stretch the quads by gently pulling upward with your right hand.

4. Repeat on the left side.

5. Make sure you are fully balanced before moving away from the wall.

Ending

Finish your stretching with deep breathing and 'Rag Doll' floppy movements.

Stretches and exercises prepared in conjunction with Noela Corby
Attribution: Some of the stretches shown above have been adapted with permission from the book
'Overcome Neck and Back Pain' by Kit Laughlin, a Fireside Book published by Simon &
Schuster. Kit Laughlin lectures at the Australian National University.

14

Song and Dance –
Talking and Walking With
Parkinson's Disease

Many of you may experience some difficulty with speech and or walking. Your voice may become softer, a stammer develop, or it may be difficult to speak the words formed in your mind. Uneven gait, freezing, festination or poor balance may inhibit your walk.

These symptoms may take some time to resolve, so here are a few 'tricks' to help you along the way.

Song

Our speech centre and song centre are quite distinctly different in our brain. If you have difficulty expressing yourself, or you stammer, sing the words in your mind before speaking, and this may improve. Or sing out loud. I did this quite often early in my Parkinson's disease journey as I had to convey instructions to my crew and my stammer was bad enough to render my conversation almost unintelligible. I performed spontaneous 'recitatives' to say what I wanted with quite good results. I'll never be an opera singer, but it worked.

Singing in private can also help improve your speech volume. Imagine you are performing in Carnegie Hall or the Sydney Opera House, and sing as loudly as you can – all your favourite songs, even if you can't remember the words; make up new words. It works! Life's an opera if you want it to be.

Dance

A common feature of Parkinson's disease is a loss of rhythm in our walk. However, if we provide an external rhythm, for instance rhythmic music or stripes on the floor, our walk will often improve.

If you have problems walking freely, sing or hum marches or jazz tunes to yourself to bring rhythm to your movement. Walk as if you *are* dancing; swing your hips, bounce lightly on your feet, let your knees flex a little. Start by playing music loudly in your home while you walk to the beat, then develop the habit of 'hearing' that rhythm in your head as you walk. This technique will often reduce freezing as well as improving the distance you can walk safely.

15

Reading

The type of literature we choose to read can significantly affect our wellbeing as our emotions are stirred by the writer or content. We have already talked about reading joke books and humorous works in the chapter on LAUGHTER, but everything we read, from the daily newspaper to periodicals to novels and non-fiction literature, can affect our attitude to life and health.

We have enormous choice in the literature we can read, and I encourage you to find works that inspire, entertain or divert you. It is not my place to tell you what you should or should not read. I believe there are no 'rules', but there are some logical thought processes that will serve us well.

The suggestions below on how to choose what to read apply equally in choosing films or television shows to watch and radio shows to listen to. Remember, we are all individuals so what entertains me may not entertain you, but literature or visual art that has a negative effect on me will probably have a negative effect on you.

- Read books and watch shows that divert you (even though you know they are fiction, and therefore 'unreal'), make you feel happy, and leave you with a good feeling at the end of the book or show. This doesn't mean it must be a 'happy ending' in the Hollywood sense, but that it leaves you with a feeling of completion and satisfaction.
- Read stories and watch shows that make you laugh, cry,

smile, cheer and/or feel proud. These may be fiction, news items, documentaries, biographies or 'soapies'.

- Avoid shows and stories that depress you, make you feel unhappy or helpless, or emphasise that you 'can't be cured and only Western medicine will find a cure if you give them lots of money'. Be selective about the news items you watch – news stories are usually biased toward sensationalism and often don't reflect the true situation and may emphasise the negative aspects of the story, or frustrate you because you 'can't do anything'. We all know bad things happen in the world, and we can only do a little to help. We don't have to spend every evening watching all the misery and generating lots of stress hormones to exacerbate our illness.

- Read or watch stories about people who triumph over difficult situations or circumstances, and know that you can do it too.

- Take time out regularly to read something light just for entertainment – fishing magazines, or car magazines or magazines about whatever your favourite pastime may be; thriller novels or detective stories or whatever type of story that takes you away from the 'real world' for a little while. It's okay to be lost in fiction sometimes.

- Set aside some time each week to read something that will help you on your pathway to wellness – a 'self-help' book, something on meditation or relaxation, a story of recovery, information about one of the therapies you're using or intend to try, or one of those wonderful little books of inspiring quotations.

You can have complete control over what you read, watch and listen to. Take this control in both hands and use it wisely to help you towards recovery.

16

Your Journal –
Your Second Friend

I talk to all my clients diagnosed with a degenerative disorder about keeping a weekly journal, or weekly notes.
This is a very simple thing to do, and a very powerful tool to
help you move toward wellness. It will take you only about
ten minutes per week to write some notes about how you
are feeling, and what has happened during the week just
past.

This is really, really important to help you see how well
you are doing, and to give your practitioners accurate information about your progress and challenges.[21]

Sometimes we develop what I like to call a 'crocodile
syndrome'. It's like this:

*One day we have to cross a swamp. While we're doing this,
we find that there are one hundred crocodiles snapping
around us, hoping to make us a meal. We're very frightened
(of course), but keep going and cross the swamp successfully.
A few weeks later, we have to cross the swamp again. The
crocodiles are still there, and we're just as frightened. We keep
thinking, 'Why are there always so many crocodiles around
whenever I have to cross the swamp?' But we don't stop to
count the crocodiles. So we don't realise that there are only
ninety crocodiles this time. The swamp is slowly getting safer
for us to cross.*

Our Parkinson's disease is like the swamp. We live with the disorder every day, so often we don't see the tiny improvements as they happen; they happen so slowly that it feels like we're standing still. But, if we keep a weekly journal, and are honest about our symptoms, feelings, and what has happened during the week, over time we will see a pattern emerging showing just how we are progressing. If I had not kept notes during my recovery, I would have given up because, so often, it seemed I was standing still or going backwards. However, when I read my notes, I could see that there were little improvements emerging, and these gave me the hope and encouragement to keep going. And now I am well.

Keep a weekly journal! Here's how to start.

Buy a notebook, or journal that you will really like to write in. Find a book with a lovely cover that feels special; one that you will like to have on the bedside table. This is going to be a record of your great adventure, so it's worth spending a few dollars on it.

Answer all the questions below as completely and as honestly as you can. You may want to copy the questions into your special notebook, or photocopy the pages in this book.

1. On what day of each week will you write notes about the week just past? ....
2. What is the date today? ....
3. How do you feel about your disorder today? Are you hopeful? Angry? Despairing? Frustrated? Challenged? Determined to get well? Be honest about your emotions and write as much as you can (three words or three pages)
   ....
   ....

....
....
....
....
....
....

4. Describe your symptoms in as much detail as possible. You have already done this for your practitioners, so it should be easy.

....
....
....
....
....
....
....
....
....
....
....

5. Ask your spouse, partner, carer or a friend to write a brief impression of you at the moment. That is, what do they see when they are with you?

....
....
....
....
....
....

Mark your 'Journal Day' in your diary or on your calendar so you will always be reminded to sit down and write your notes.

***Keep in mind that this is a TEN MINUTES PER WEEK
DEDICATION TO YOUR RECOVERY.***

Now, that wasn't too hard, was it? Whenever you see any
health practitioner, read your journal before your visit and
either take notes about questions to be asked and points to
be noted, or take your journal with you and use that as a
memory jogger for what you want to talk to your practitioner about. This will help you and your practitioner to
understand just how well you are doing.

Ten minutes each week is all it takes.

17

Other Ways to Help Yourself

Many of us who develop Parkinson's disease have spent most of our lives believing that what we do represents what we are worth, so we concentrate on work or 'duties', often neglecting ourselves, our relationships and families in the process. Often we accept adult levels of responsibility in childhood because that is what we think is expected of us. As we move into adulthood, 'responsible habits' may become ingrained in our psyche, creating frustration at their restraint, guilt if we don't live up to expectations, and fatigue from such unrelenting pressure. We may be inhibited from expressing playfulness and joy.

It's time to change. Treating ourselves with love is just as important as treating others with love. Doing things that make us feel joyful, happy, or at peace with ourselves can have a positive and healthy effect on our body.

We've talked about laughter, reading, watching shows and exercising. There are many other activities that might suit you, and it is good to put aside some time each week to participate in a hobby, team sport or a form of art that gives you a feeling of achievement, companionship and relaxed activity.

Here are a few ideas. The list is certainly not exhaustive, and I encourage you to look about your community to see what novel and entertaining activities are available to help you feel happy with life.

- Dancing: Did you go to church dances, or school socials? Did you enjoy the feeling of whirling and sliding around the floor with a companion in your arms? Start again. There are lots of dance opportunities now; dance studios often have public times where you can just go and dance for a small fee, some communities run regular Saturday night dances, or get a few friends together in your family room for some old time dancing. If you have never been a dancer, this might be a good time to start; take some private lessons to learn a few basic steps, then join a group class and enjoy the company. Dancing is excellent exercise too.

- Movement Classes: There are many forms of creative movement, often offered at Community Centres. Movement to music, expressing yourself through movement, or simply moving with an instructor can help you become freer in your mobility.

- Acting: Join a local drama group or musical theatre and 'lose' yourself in another character. Help with backdrops and sets, or work as a stagehand. You'll enjoy the company of others and the achievement of producing a good show.

- Painting: Can be a wonderful way to express your deepest feelings without having to find words. If you have never painted before, find a local class and go for it. You don't have to compete with anyone, or meet any 'quality standards'; just use the medium, colours and techniques that express what YOU feel.

- Pottery and Clay Modelling: A fabulous way to get your hands dirty and ending up with something to show for it. Working with clay can be relaxing, fun and satisfying.

- Working with wood: Haven't got a shed at home? Find a local woodworking class and build something useful for

YOU – a new bookcase, stool, table or whatever. Timber is warm and welcoming and you might just make a masterpiece.

- Gardening: Perhaps you haven't been a gardener before. Now is a good time to dig in the soil, discover new plants and have the satisfaction of watching your 'babies' grow. You might like to start a vegetable garden to give yourself the gift of organically grown, loved food. Or grow some herbs to add flavour to your food. If a large garden is too much for you, start with a few pot plants on the front verandah. Flowers, herbs and even vegies do well in pots and give a real sense of achievement as you nurture their growth. I grow some lovely roses and native shrubs in pots with minimum effort, and really enjoy it.
- Discussion Groups: There are many groups meeting to discuss books, films, ideas and all sorts of other important or unimportant matters. Find one that includes people with a good sense of humour, and where the discussion isn't too serious. This is relaxation, remember.

Look around your local community for activities that you find interesting, will inspire you to take part regularly and will teach you some new skills. Choose activities that extend your physical capabilities just a little. Above all, have fun!

18

Sexuality and Parkinson's Disease

If we are in a loving relationship, sex may play an important role as a means of expressing that love. As our Parkinson's disease symptoms develop, we may find that we lose interest in sex, or become impotent.

This subject is surrounded by confusion, ignorance, frustration, embarrassment and silence. Most health practitioners feel unprepared to discuss sexual relationships as it is not included in our training. Patients are often embarrassed to speak to a relative stranger about such private matters, and may feel humiliated by their inability to enjoy sexual intercourse with their partner. Partners may be frustrated and feel rejected, not understanding how such a profound change in sexual ability can occur in someone whose other Parkinson's disease symptoms may seem relatively mild.

Sexual behaviour is, in part, controlled by our hypothalamus. This control centre has been profoundly affected by the long-term, unresolved stress (whatever it was) that began our journey into the expression of Parkinson's disease symptoms. This is why sexual function may be changed in many diagnosed with Parkinson's disease, along with appetite, thirst and temperature control.

The effect of developing Parkinson's disease on sexual ability and desire varies enormously from person to person. Some may simply lose interest; some may have a normal or heightened desire, but become impotent; others may find their libido and potency fluctuating widely from day to day, without any apparent pattern or reason. Whatever the effect for us, these changes undoubtedly affect our relationship and our sense of self-esteem.

A small, but important sub-group in this discussion consists of men who have been diagnosed with Parkinson's disease following prostate surgery – usually Trans Urethral Radical Prostatectomy. The trauma of the surgery and anaesthetic seems to be the final trigger for their body, and Parkinson's disease symptoms occur within weeks or a few months of the procedure, often accompanied by incontinence and impotence as a result of the surgery.

I am not a trained sex therapist, nor a qualified counsellor dealing with relationship issues. However, I experienced enormous changes in my libido and potency during my journey with Parkinson's disease, and found some solutions. Since commencing practice in 1998, I have spoken with many patients about this part of their life, and worked with them to find answers that suited them and their partners. The suggestions below are borne from my personal experience during my illness and in practice. At all times, it is wise and helpful to seek the assistance of an experienced and caring practitioner.

- *Talk about it*: The most important part in any relationship is communication. There are many ways we communicate non-verbally but, when circumstances change, as in illness, we need to talk to our partner and make sure we both understand what is going on, and how we feel. If you lose interest in sex, or find sexual intercourse difficult, tell your partner and ask them to be patient and help you. Ask your partner how they feel and discuss ways of expressing your love outside of sexual intercourse.

- *Change the way you have intercourse*: If you are experiencing desire with impotence, experiment with different ways to stimulate your body. Slow down and enjoy longer and gentler foreplay; enjoy some sexy talk during the hours before bed to get the idea in your head and body; exchange jokes about sex and laugh together; use gentle, patient touching to improve blood flow and stimulation. You may find that some new positions, less physically demanding, give more satisfaction and less frustration. Above all, be very patient with yourself and your partner.

- *Touch each other more*: Loving touch is one of the best 'turn ons' there is. I don't mean sexual touch, but the gentle touch that says 'I love you, right at this moment'. Rub your fingertips gently on your partner's shoulder as you pass, stroke their hair (or head) gently, give them a 'butterfly kiss' on the cheek or ear, very gently stroke the inside of their knee for just a second or two, or hold their hand and very gently stroke their fingers. Frequent, gentle, loving touching is much more successful than meeting in bed and expecting to 'perform' immediately.

- *Talk to your health practitioner*: There are many herbal, homeopathic and flower essence remedies that may help you with both libido and potency. I strongly suggest you avoid drugs such as Tadalafil (Cialis), Sildenafil (Viagra), Vardenafil (Levitra) and similar, as they may exacerbate your Parkinson's disease symptoms. In practice, I have found that, while these drugs may enable sexual intercourse at a particular moment, they do nothing to address the underlying cause, and may have long-term effects that are very undesirable. I have used a number of herbal preparations successfully, (especially for erectile dysfunction in

men and hormone imbalance in women) plus homeopathic support. Flower essences can often assist with
emotional and intellectual barriers to successful intercourse.

- *Talk to a counsellor*: If you find that it is difficult to talk to
  your partner without becoming overcome with emotion
  or confused, seek help from an empathetic counsellor. Go
  together to some meetings and talk through your feelings
  openly and honestly, knowing you will not be judged in
  any way.

- *Remember it may not be the Parkinson's disease*: Sometimes
  developing a serious disorder like Parkinson's disease
  brings back to our mind forgotten memories of long ago,
  feelings of anger and frustration from childhood, or fear
  imposed on us by others. These feelings may dramatically affect our sexual performance. Talk to your counsellor
  about what you are really feeling NOW, and you may
  find your sexual difficulties diminish significantly.

- *Enjoy what you have*: If you are in a loving, supportive
  relationship, congratulations! You have opportunities to
  talk with, hold, sleep beside, go out with and have adven-
  tures with someone who loves you on a daily basis. Not
  everyone has that privilege. Walking hand in hand, lying
  in each others arms and talking, pottering around the
  garden together, watching the sunset while holding
  hands, writing poetry for each other and so many other
  beautiful activities are wonderful ways to say 'I love you'.
  Explore what you have, and find new ways to enjoy each
  other. You are very lucky people.

My personal experience is that, during my journey with
Parkinson's disease, on the rare occasions I was lucky enough
to have a loving partner with me, we could enjoy fun together,

explore our bodies in new and exciting ways, and patiently stimulate my body to respond eventually. If we approached the process as a new adventure each time, a process of discovery and humour, we were able to celebrate being together with very little frustration.

If you are experiencing changes in your sexual desires or abilities, remember that your greatest help, and best friend is the person closest to you.

Section Three

There's Help Out There For You

If you have decided to accept responsibility for your health and take control of your journey to wellness, you are probably already participating in many of the activities and life changes I have spoken about in the preceding chapters.

The good news is that you don't have to do it all yourself. There are therapies and practitioners who can and will help you to improve your health.

The next section deals with many types of medicine; conservative Western medicine and so-called complementary medicine. I have given you my frank opinion of each modality and information about how and why it works or doesn't work. In the end, you are the only person who can truly tell whether a particular therapy is good for you.

Beware of practitioners, sales people or manufacturers who make outlandish claims of 'cure'; there is no cure, even though we can recover. Be equally wary of those practitioners who say there is no hope of recovery; they are simply seeking to impose their ignorance on you.

Above all, enquire, ask questions and be sure you feel 'right' before embarking on any course of treatment.

19

Medication

Your neurologist is the best person to advise you about which medication is likely to give you the greatest benefits. If you choose to use Western medication as part of your journey to better health, seek advice from your chosen neurologist, and be prepared to ask a lot of questions, and keep on asking until you get answers that satisfy you. Then spend time in considering how YOU feel about their advice.

The information on Western medication contained in this book is gleaned from drug guides, medical journals, other medical books as shown, and my experience in clinic since 1998.

There are a number of medicines now available to help you control Parkinson's disease symptoms while you are working to reverse the disease process. Prior to 1967, the only medications available were amantadine and some anticholinergic drugs.[21] The way amantadine works is still not really understood, but it is thought it may enhance dopamine receptor activity and/or slow the reuptake of dopamine in the brain.[1] Anticholinergic drugs reduce the amount of available acetylcholine, thus increasing, in relative terms, the amount of dopamine available.

Both types of medication have limited benefits and produce a wide range of distressing side effects.

The introduction of levodopa drugs in the 1960's

brought a revolution in the treatment of Parkinson's disease. For the first time, many people diagnosed with this distressing disorder were able to gain real relief from many of their symptoms and resume 'normal' life for a significant period. Levodopa is the precursor to dopamine and is normally produced in our brain, then converted into dopamine through a fairly complex process. It is thought (though not yet fully proven) that the levodopa contained in commonly prescribed levodopa drugs is converted to dopamine and utilised in our brain in a similar way to naturally produced levodopa.

The levodopa drugs used in the USA, Canada and Australia are Sinemet, Madopar, Atamet, Larodopa, Apo-levocarb, Nu-levocarb and Kinson. All are packaged with a decarboxylase inhibitor that reduces the amount of levodopa absorbed before crossing into the brain. Before these decarboxylase inhibitors were added, much of the levodopa taken orally was absorbed into tissue before reaching the brain, exacerbating the side effects of nausea, and necessitating a much higher dose each time to gain reasonable benefit. Sinemet, Atamet, Larodopa, Apo-levocarb, Nu-levocarb and Kinson are packaged with Carbidopa while Madopar is packaged with Benserazide.[1]

Your neurologist may ask you to commence one brand of drug, then change to another if the effect is not what you desire. The difference may be simply the different decarboxylase inhibitor used, as we can respond well to one, but not the other.

Your neurologist may also suggest you start your treatment by taking a dopamine agonist only. Common dopamine agonists are bromocriptine (Parlodel or Kripton), pergolide (Permax) and cabergoline (Cabaser).[45] These drugs do not supply extra dopamine, but are thought to stimulate dopamine receptors to accept more of the available dopamine.[1,45] While there may be some advantages in beginning your treatment this way, my experience indicates that the most effective drug treatment is a combination of levodopa and dopamine agonist, or levodopa alone for some significant period.

Sometimes older, anticholinergic drugs are used in combination with levodopa drugs to try to gain relief of specific symptoms. Anticholinergic drugs most commonly used are benzhexol (Artane), benztropine (Cogentin), biperiden (Akineton), orphenadrine (Disipal) and procyclidine (Kemadrin).[45] Your neurologist will explain reasons for prescribing these drugs if they are considered necessary.

Selegiline (Elderpryl, Selgene) is a monoamine oxidase B inhibitor that reduces the rate of breakdown of dopamine in the brain, thus making relatively more dopamine available. Your neurologist may prescribe one of these drugs in conjunction with levodopa to keep the dose of levodopa required to a minimum.[1,45]

COMT inhibitors block the action of another chemical (catechol-O-methyl transferase) that breaks down dopamine in the brain. Tolecapone (Tasmar) was the first drug of this type released, but was withdrawn in Australia, and used with caution elsewhere from 1998 after reports of three deaths from hepatitis following use of the drug. Another COMT inhibitor, Entacapone (Comtan), was released shortly after and is commonly prescribed in conjunction with levodopa drugs.[45]

My experience since 1998 indicates that levodopa drugs are still the most effective in reducing the symptoms of Parkinson's disease. Dopamine agonists, MAO B inhibitors and COMT inhibitors help some people, but their effect is incremental and there are many people who do not benefit from these additional drugs.

Preserving the usefulness of l'dopa

When taking any levodopa drug (Kinson, Madopar, Atamet, Larodopa, Apo-levocarb, Nu-levocarb or Sinemet) it is very important to protect yourself against long-term damage caused by the breakdown of dopamine in the brain. If protective measures are taken, your levodopa drugs will be more effective for a longer period, and you may be able to stay on a lower dose than otherwise.

When l'dopa is converted to dopamine in the brain, the dopamine is utilised and broken down to a number of different chemical compounds; a few of these metabolites (breakdown products) may be harmful to brain cells. Some metabolites such as 6 hydroxy-dopa, other quinones and free radicals are thought to both damage cells and slow the conversion of l'dopa to dopamine. Our best protection against these effects is consumption of therapeutic doses of vitamin C and other antioxidants such as vitamin E, Coenzyme Q10, etc, and hydrating our cells. These supplements and hydration are discussed in earlier chapters.

A very important metabolite of dopamine use is homocysteine. This chemical, when in excess, is implicated in a number of degenerative processes including heart disease and neurological disorders. However, we can slow this process down by reducing the amount of homocysteine hanging around quite easily.

If you are taking any l'dopa drug, always take the following supplements:

Folic acid	500 mcg daily
Vitamin C	2000 mg twice daily
Vitamin B complex	1 high potency tablet daily.

You may find it more convenient to take one of the 'anti homocysteine' preparations available from some naturopaths and health food stores. Most Anti-Homocysteine Factor preparations contain Folic Acid, plus synergistic elements to increase its effectiveness, including vitamin B6. I suggest that you take vitamin C as noted above if you use a preparation like this.

Prior to the packaging of levodopa with a decarboxylase inhibitor, vitamin B6 (pyridoxine hydrochloride) inhibited the absorption and utilisation of the drug. However, studies have shown that it is now quite safe to take vitamin B6 with Levodopa drugs as there is no change in absorption rates.[1]

Dosage

When prescribing levodopa drugs, most neurologists ask you to start with a small dose (50 mg or 100 mg) three times daily, increasing the dose by 50 or 100 mg each few days or each week until a reasonable reduction in symptoms is achieved. Most will say nothing about taking Folic Acid, vitamin C or any other supplement.

In my experience, it is better to stay on a very low dose (50 mg three times daily) for six to eight weeks before increasing the dose. Little, if any, benefit will be felt for the first three or four weeks but, after that, there will most likely be a gradual increase in benefit. You may find that you can maintain this low dose for many months, or need only a very small increase in the amount taken.

Increases in dosage should also be maintained for at least four weeks before any change. Changes in Parkinson's disease symptoms happen very slowly, and our response to both Western and complementary medicine is no different – it happens slowly.

The disadvantage of using a low dose of levodopa over a

long period is that symptom relief will take much longer to happen. But the advantage is that you can stay on a low dose for much longer, thus reducing the damaging effects of the drug, decreasing the need for other drugs to be taken in conjunction with your levodopa, and giving your body a much greater chance of reversing your symptoms.

Time of dose

Your doctor may insist on you taking your dose of levodopa at a set time each day without variation. You may find, however, that your response to the medication, and your need for the next dose, varies from day to day. This can occur with changes in activity, stress levels, foods eaten and even weather conditions.

You may decide to spend some extra time in bed on weekends, or perhaps you are on holidays and starting your day more slowly. At these times, you may decide to take your first dose for the day a little later. Your need for the second and third dose may vary by one or two hours, and you are the best judge of this.

I suggest that you, initially, take your levodopa strictly to the timetable set out by your doctor. Observe closely how long it takes for each dose to have a beneficial effect, how long it lasts, and the signs that your medication is wearing off (your Journal will be very helpful for this). Once you understand your individual response, you are in the best position to judge when you need another dose to support you through the next few hours.

A number of my clients enjoy using their medication in this way. On busy days, they may take their medicine every four to five hours. On easier days, the first dose may last up to six hours, the second dose for the rest of the afternoon and, if they are not doing much in the evening, they may decide not to take the third dose. This works well for them and preserves the usefulness of the medication over a longer period.

Varying the dose

Many clients also find that they can vary the dose taken a little to allow for variations in activity and stress levels. For instance, you may normally take 50 mg three times daily. On Tuesdays, however, you have a particularly busy day and experience some extra stress during business hours. So, each Tuesday, you take 100 mg for your second dose just to give you that extra support during the stressful period.

It works! Many people with Parkinson's disease have taken control of their medication and are using it in a way that best suits their individual needs.

L'dopa medication may be of assistance in relieving your Parkinson's disease symptoms. However, it will not slow the degeneration causing your symptoms, nor help you reverse your symptoms. Make use of this medicine to give you the level of support you need to help you function in the most normal way possible, while utilising the lowest possible dose to preserve its usefulness over a longer period.

Always inform your doctor of any decisions you make about your medication. Many will support your right to make these decisions. If your doctor is not supportive, or becomes abusive (and, unfortunately, some are abusive), find another doctor.[21] There are wonderful supportive and understanding General Practitioners and neurologists around; it is up to us to find them.

Beyond
There is strength in silence
There is strength in patience

There is strength in wisdom
There is strength in peace
There is strength in unconditional love
There is strength in going beyond the convention and resisting the temptation to blindly follow what they say you must do
There is strength in following your heart and the guidance of God for what you know is true
There is strength in all these things for they are the very things that bond us to one another and set us free
And with them there is great strength in you and me

Jill Marjama-Lyons, M.D.[21]
Neurologist, Florida, USA

20

Bodywork

There are many forms of excellent bodywork available that can bring comfort and assist mobility for those with Parkinson's disease. Many forms of bodywork will bring comfort simply because we are receiving loving touch from a caring practitioner; some will generate chemical reactions (eg. producing endorphins – 'natural painkillers') that provide physical comfort; a few modalities will bring positive therapeutic effects to our lives.

During my journey with Parkinson's disease, I experimented with a number of bodywork modalities – massage of various types, Craniosacral therapy, Feldenkrais, Reflexology, Osteopathy and Bowen Therapy.[46] I found advantages and disadvantages with most and it became clear that the most important component in delivering the therapy was the practitioner. If my therapist was of the type who simply 'sells' their therapy or 'processes' their clients, then I rarely gained any benefit and often felt much worse. If, on the other hand, the therapist showed they cared about me and my journey, took time to understand what I and my body needed in the way of duration and intensity of treatment, I always gained some benefit.

It became clear, and this has been confirmed by my experience in practice, that people with Parkinson's disease need VERY GENTLE bodywork, no matter how robust or confident we may appear. This makes sense when we consider that an underlying condition with Parkinson's disease is cell fragility. If our cell membranes are fragile, they need gentle persuasion to resume their 'normal' function and resilience; hard or rough bodywork is likely to have an adverse effect.

After trying many forms of bodywork during my journey with Parkinson's disease, I found that Bowen Therapy, combined with the Aqua Hydration Formulas and self-help activities, brought the greatest benefit.[46] However, many forms of bodywork can, and do help those with Parkinson's disease, and it is good to try any that seem right to you; I must emphasise again, however, that your therapist must treat you with gentleness, respect and compassion.

My observations below are borne from personal experience, clinical observation and research with many experienced practitioners.

Bowen therapy; pumping water

Bowen therapy is very gentle bodywork developed by Thomas Bowen in Geelong, Australia, during the late 1940's and early 1950's. It consists of gentle movements across muscles, tendons and ligaments to relieve pain, spasm and stiffness of movement.

Tom Bowen was intuitive in his diagnosis and could often correct dysfunction with a single treatment or, at the most, three. He was extremely busy, often seeing fourteen patients per hour; this equated to approximately 11,000 patients per year. He successfully treated all sorts of conditions ranging from intractable pain, muscle spasm, sporting injuries, respiratory problems to arthritis as well as other chronic disorders.[47,48]

Most Bowen therapists today do not see patients at the rate that Tom Bowen did during his busiest years. While some therapists may have two rooms in operation at once, many see one patient only at a time and spend from half an hour to one-and-a-half hours in treatment.

A Bowen therapy session consists of light movements across the bellies of muscles, tendons or ligaments, then pauses for two or more minutes to allow the patient's body to make adjustments.

There are a number of hypotheses concerning the way Bowen therapy works. Current research indicates that there are probably two major effects created by the therapist's moves during a Bowen therapy session. The first is the movement of water through the fascia, and movement of fascia.[29] Fascia is a protein substance, like the white of an egg, made up of proteoglycans and glycosaminoglycans, contains collagen and reticulin fibres, and fills all the apparent spaces in our body between organs, muscles, bones, tendons and ligaments, and the brain (the dura) – the 'gaps' between the various parts of our body that appear separate in anatomy charts.[29] Fascia carries fluids, immune system cells, and other elements vital to our wellbeing. During times of illness, injury, fatigue or stress, fascia can become 'cooked', like an egg white, and firmly attached to the muscle or bone it surrounds, and no longer allow free movement of fluid and nutrients. This can create discomfort, stiffness or pain and inhibit our return to wellness.[29]

The second major effect of a Bowen therapy treatment is a movement of electrical energy throughout the body. This can be thought of as electrical current, Qi, Prana or life-energy depending on the philosophy you're coming from. However we view it, it is vital to have a balanced electrical energy flow throughout our bodies for us to feel well and satisfied with our life. The moves in a Bowen therapy session serve to remove blockages, correct imbalances, and restore free flow of electrical energy over the whole body even though the moves are made only at specific points. This is similar to the work done in acupuncture or acupressure.

My adventure with Bowen therapy began in 1996 when I read an article about the therapy in the International Journal of Alternative and Complementary Medicine.[47] I had never heard of Bowen therapy before, let alone had any Bowen treatment. Despite my ignorance, I intuitively knew that I needed to train as a Bowen therapist, and set about finding a teacher. It took many months before I was able to find a class which would accept me and, in July 1997, I trained with Rick Loader. This began a real love affair with Bowen therapy. Almost immediately, I transferred most of my massage clients to Bowen therapy because I could obtain such great success using this therapy rather than traditional massage. Despite my training however, I did not have formal treatment from a Bowen therapist until late in 1997 when I went back to Rick for treatment on my frozen right shoulder.

I started treating people with Parkinson's disease using Bowen therapy and Aqua Hydration Formulas in the second half of 1998. This was very much an experiment because I had used a large number of therapies to obtain my own recovery. However, intuitively and intellectually, I believed that Bowen therapy and hydration were the major therapies instrumental in my full recovery.

Two years after my first training, I completed a Neuro-structural Integration Technique course, and was amazed at the power of this more advanced Bowen Therapy. Since then, I have treated people displaying the symptoms of Parkinson's disease, Multiple Sclerosis, Multi-System Atrophy, Motor Neurone Disease, Spasmodic Torticollis, Lupus, Ankylosing Spondylitis and a variety of other degenerative disorders, using the combination of Aqua Hydration Formulas and Bowen Therapy, plus other therapies as required.

Bowen therapy is very powerful treatment for pain, injury and a number of illnesses. However, I have found in the treatment of neurological disorders, that it works best with the Aqua Hydration Formulas and some accompanying therapies described in other chapters. While some improvement in Parkinson's disease symptoms can be obtained by using only Bowen therapy, the results are generally slow and unsatisfying. Using the hydration effect of Aqua Hydration Formulas, plus the hydrating and balancing effect of Bowen therapy is very powerful medicine indeed. All those who have come to me with Parkinson's disease and persisted with this therapy have made great steps forward in returning to health.

Any Bowen therapist treating patients with neurological disorders needs to remember that the pain and stiffness displayed by their patient is neurological in origin – not physical. Therefore, the therapy needs to be gentle and balancing, despite the often asymmetrical nature of the symptoms displayed. Treatment which is too firm or asymmetrical in approach can be detrimental to your progress, as well as causing unnecessary pain.

The timing of treatments is important also. Many therapists try to see their Parkinson's disease patients frequently in the hope of gaining significant result within a short period. My experience indicates that this is rarely satisfactory. Occasionally, I see patients weekly in order to help them over a difficult patch – for instance, when they are reducing medication or experiencing extra stress in their lives. Generally, however, I find that **treatments every two weeks** work well.

Remember, **RECOVERING FROM PARKINSON'S DISEASE TAKES AT LEAST THREE YEARS OR MORE**. It is very important to establish a supportive, comforting relationship with your Bowen therapist so you can both enjoy and learn from this exciting, challenging journey.

If you are a person suffering from Parkinson's disease, Bowen therapy can open the way to freeing you from many inhibiting issues from the past. **Counselling, kinesiology, hypnotherapy and/or Flower Essences** are often wonderful accompaniments to this work and you may want to work with therapists who are prepared to join you on this adventure.

There are a number of interpretations of Tom Bowen's principles of healing that are now available for study or treatment. Bowtech, Bowen Essentials, Neurostructural Integration Technique, Fascial Kinetics, Smart Bowen and International School of Bowen Therapy courses are available throughout Australia, while Bowtech, Neurostructural Integration Technique (NST) and International School of Bowen Therapy are taught in many countries. There are practitioners, colleges and associations around the world.

Information for Bowen practitioners and therapists

Show this section to your chosen Bowen therapist and ask them to read it thoroughly before commencing work together.

Neurological disorders are difficult to treat for three reasons:

1. *The skeletal and muscular dysfunctions we observe are neurological in origin and do not respond to Bowen in the same way as injuries and skeletal imbalances.*
2. *The symptoms occur as a result of damage to, or destruction of, brain cells over a wide area. Therefore, long-term or permanent improvement can only result from repair or regeneration of these brain cells.*
3. *Repair, and consequent resolution of symptoms, takes a very long time, and cannot be hurried.*

Each Bowen session serves a number of purposes. Each of these purposes is equally important, and it is vital that we do not concentrate solely on the physical manifestations of the disease.

Each time you see your Parkinson's disease patient, you bring to them the following gifts:

1. *Contact with a professional health practitioner who believes they can become well.*
2. *Contact with a health practitioner who gives them time to speak and listens to what they have to say.*
3. *The knowledge that they are complete, beautiful human beings, worthy of your undivided care and attention.*
4. *The healing touch of Bowen Therapy.*
5. *The certainty that they will receive the comfort you give them on a regular basis.*
6. *An assessment of their current condition and progress over time.*

Even though there are a number of Bowen Therapy schools teaching different interpretations of Tom Bowen's work, all are valid; all can help people with Parkinson's disease move toward health. There are, however, principals of treatment which should be observed closely:

- ***If it hurts, it's too hard***. *The purpose of Bowen Therapy in treating neurological disorders is to move and hydrate fascia, balance energy and encourage regeneration/ reactivation of brain cells. Therefore, the therapy does not need to be hard or deep. In my experience, digging too deeply into muscles that are rigid, locked and painful is counter-productive; it causes the muscles to become even more rigid, creates pain, and operates on a physical, rather than a neurological level.*

- **All treatment should be symmetrical, except for the coccyx move, specific neuro balance moves and extraordinary circumstances.** *Two of the purposes of using Bowen Therapy are to encourage symmetrical energy within the brain and symmetry of physical movement. Therefore, the therapy needs to be symmetrical. The coccyx move is, of its nature, asymmetrical and serves to promote symmetry of energy along and around the spine, as does the Advanced NST Neuro Balance move. Occasionally, there is a need to treat a specific asymmetrical condition such as a frozen shoulder or asymmetrical back pain. Asymmetrical treatment is appropriate here, but it needs to be understood that this is simply treating the physical symptoms of a neurological condition.*
- **Bowen Therapy can't do it alone.** *It is tempting to think that persistent use of Bowen Therapy will eventually create a healing pathway without recourse to any other therapy. In my experience, this is not possible with Parkinson's disease. Bowen Therapy is a critical, integral part of a synergistic recovery programme. It helps give mobility and peace as well as the benefits described above.*
- **Many people with Parkinson's disease are old, frail and rigid. All are very sensitive.** *It is very important to move each muscle group or limb only as much as is comfortable for the patient. The rigidity, pain and slowness of movement shown by our patients is neurological in origin and we must be patient in 're-educating the brain' to allow freedom of movement. It has been my personal experience that attempting to create freedom of movement by challenging rigidity is painful, depressing and inclined to set us back or discourage us from trying to get well.*

Bowen Therapy is one way to gain a real appreciation of the progress toward health each person is making.

Is there a standard protocol?

Following the first one or two treatments, I find it most effective to give my clients a 'complete' treatment at each visit. I do not intend to describe specific moves to use during any one treatment, rather I wish to set down principles of treatment I have found to be effective over the last five years. Because each interpretation of Tom Bowen's work names the moves differently, I will give general descriptions only.

Each practitioner should assess his or her client on each visit as you do now. Treatments may need to be varied from a set routine because of particular stresses, accidents or changes in your client's condition.

On the first two visits, I suggest that basic moves only be used covering the back, neck and legs. On the second visit, it may be useful to introduce the TMJ move if your client is robust enough. This can assist with balance and mobility.

From the third visit, I like to do a 'complete' Bowen treatment each time. This includes the basic back moves (sometimes freeing the erector spinae muscles) and, often, extra hip moves where mobility is a problem, plus sacrum and hamstrings while prone. I almost always include a 'neuro balance move' (advanced NST) and often, when supine, the pelvic moves including psoas. In the supine position, I use abdominal/respiratory moves, neck, knee, ankle, shoulder, elbow and wrist (carpal tunnel) and, almost invariably, the TMJ. I work slowly and very lightly, with variable pauses, to let each client relax and gain full benefit from the treatment.

I also incorporate a form of Yin Tuina on the feet and a specific cranial move. Information on these moves is available from Return To Stillness.

If you are skilled in any other form of foot or cranial work, you may wish to incorporate some individual moves into your

There's Help Out There For You

routine. However, people receiving basic Bowen Therapy from a loving practitioner who uses a **very light** touch make good progress. I cannot emphasise enough how important it is to use **EXTREMELY LIGHT** touch. Firmness of touch will only result in discomfort and aggravation of symptoms. The MAXI-MUM weight I suggest for any Bowen Therapy move, is the pressure you would willingly apply to your closed eye without causing discomfort. This equates to **less than five grams** of weight.

Following testing during 2001, we have been able to esti-mate that Bowen Therapy constitutes about 25% of the physical recovery process. It works synergistically with the Aqua Hydration Formulas which do about 60% of the work. So Bowen is vitally important to people recovering from neurologi-cal disorders, but will give greatest benefits when used with hydration therapy.

Remember, you are the practitioner your client sees most often. Therefore, you have a unique opportunity to join them on their great adventure. I encourage you to participate fully and enjoy the experience.

Please contact me at my practice if you have any questions about Bowen Therapy for neurological disorders, or wish to dis-cuss the progress of your client.

A significant symptom of Parkinson's disease is muscular stiffness, rigidity and pain. During my long prodromal period of over thirty years, I had sought therapies other than Bowen Therapy to alleviate and/or cure these symptoms which were progressing slowly.

Chiropractic seemed to be a logical choice as most of my pain and stiffness was blamed on posture, work injury or car accidents. I persisted with chiropractic treatment for over 20 years with little success. Certainly, I almost always gained some symptomatic relief after each treatment, but it did not 'hold'. Within two or three days, the symptoms would return, rapidly reaching the pre-treatment severity. I sometimes had three or four treatments close together to try and consolidate benefits, but the result was the same – a rapid return to pre-treatment status. A number of chiropractors told me that I was a 'lifetime chiropractic patient'.

Massage. I tried massage on several occasions over the years and enjoyed the experience but, as with chiropractic, gained only short-term alleviation of pain. Neither massage nor chiropractic could do more than lessen the pain level for a short time; they could not take it away.

Early in my adventure, I was given fortnightly **deep massages** by a colleague. We theorised that the significant muscle movement which occurs during massage would ease rigidity and enhance the work done by CST. We were wrong. While I felt invigorated and encouraged after each massage, my body rebelled within twenty four hours by giving me dreadful cramps and pain in all the muscle groups massaged. I persisted for a few weeks hoping that my body would get used to the procedure as I was in the habit of 'making my body obey me', but had to give up as the pain was too great.

I later received some gentle **relaxation massages** from another colleague. While these did little for my rigidity and pain, they definitely increased my sense of wellbeing and helped me reconnect my poor old body with the 'real person hiding inside'.

Greg Morling, National President of the Australian Association of Massage Therapists, has written a useful article on massaging Parkinson's disease patients and emphasises the need to be aware of the frailty of the Parkinsonian body.[49] I am convinced that there is a significant place for **careful, aware massage** in the treatment of Parkinson's disease.

Massage will not cure any of the Parkinsonian symptoms, but will enhance the ability of the Person With Parkinson's to pursue their goal of recovery.

Acupuncture and **cupping** were also tried at various times and were successful in easing specific symptoms at specific sites, but, again, brought no long-term relief.

By the time of my crisis in August 1995, I had been in escalating pain, with associated rigidity and stiffness, for over thirty years. (In fact, in June 1998, I celebrated my first pain-free birthday in 35 years).

My referral to a **Craniosacral Therapist** by my naturopath was fortuitous and a real breakthrough in my health. My therapist's opinion that all my physical symptoms at the time were related to the head injury sustained in childhood modified her approach to my treatment. The CT and MRI scans had eliminated the possibilities of MS, stroke, infarct, lesion and tumour, so the symptomatic diagnosis of Parkinson's disease seemed logical. The only contentious issue was whether the Parkinsonian symptoms were caused by my head injury or were idiopathic as was believed by my neurologist.

The head injury was a flattening of my skull on the left side involving most of the left temporal bone. As my birth was considered 'normal', it is likely that this was caused by frequent and/or sustained impact before the age of five. In the light of my hypothesis for the development of Parkinson's disease, this is simply another symptom, but it had a profound effect on my wellbeing.

My therapist used gentle osteopathic and massage techniques to ease the rigidity in muscles with direct influence on the cranial structure, plus any others causing pain. While techniques varied from visit to visit, the process did not vary. Julie would first ease rigid muscles, then work on the cranium. This, of course, makes sense as muscles directly or indirectly attaching to the cranial structure will influence cranial 'stress' levels, while cranial health and fascial integrity will influence almost the entire body.[50,51]

Craniosacral Therapy (CST), like all 'energy-based' bodywork techniques, is a comprehensive, holistic therapy that can be used as a stand-alone therapy or in conjunction with any other allopathic, alternative or complementary modality. My therapist was happy for me to experiment with any other therapy while she was treating me. She said, 'You are in charge. You are your own best doctor'.

There were three major aims as a focus for my CST:

- free up the suture lines and allow normal movement again;
- improve the flow of cerebrospinal fluid (CSF) throughout the central nervous system (CNS);
- improve the vascularity, plasticity and vital strength of the bones in my skull damaged by repeated impacts – especially the left temporal bone.

Conventional wisdom accepts that it is normal for the skull's suture lines to become immovable in some adults, especially older adults. Craniosacral Therapists disagree. In their view, the sutures need to remain free to make extremely small, but palpable movements in order to allow the CSF to flow freely. The sutures can be felt to move in a rhythmic way, independent of cardiac and respiratory rhythms, which coincides with the production and flow of CSF. If the sutures are completely immovable, the movement of CSF is inhibited, causing nerve dysfunction.

The brain is covered by the dura mater, part of the continuous fascia that surrounds all subcutaneous parts of our body. Lymph and cerebrospinal fluid spread throughout the craniosacral system via channels in the fascia.[52] Inhibition of movement in the skull's sutures also impedes flow of CSF through the fascia. As this is continuous throughout the body, this inhibition can have detrimental effects far from the cause. Areas of particular concern are the tentorium cerebelli and falx cerebri, folds in the dura mater that extend into major brain fissures – the cerebrum/cerebellum fissure and the longitudinal fissure respectively. These folds may be damaged during birth (too fast, too long in the birth canal, or forceps delivery) and are particularly far reaching in their effect on all body systems.[52] Injuries similar to birthing injuries are likely to cause similar detrimental effects.

My therapist also discovered that the left temporal bone of my skull felt solid and immovable like concrete, unlike the slightly flexible feel of normal living bone. In her opinion, this could only have been the result of repeated impacts against something solid.*

For over two years, during fortnightly visits, my therapist worked assiduously to restore free flow of CSF, ease my rigidity and pain, enhance the physical improvements resulting from other therapies, and bring some 'life' back to my left temporal bone. Her care enabled me to keep on working during my journey.

Craniosacral Therapy continues to be a nurturing and comforting therapy for many of my clients who often alternate CST treatments with Bowen Therapy on a weekly basis.

Feldenkrais is a bodywork modality developed by Moshe Feldenkrais to facilitate the 'integration of the skeletal, developmental, environmental and neuromuscular systems'.[53] It

---

*In August 1998, a Physiotherapist made similar observations about my left temporal bone. She was puzzled by the lack of 'life' and response felt in that bone, in contrast to the other bones of my skull.

offers a framework in which the patterns of movement, thought and feeling can be explored.[53]

Moshe Feldenkrais said of his method, 'What I'm after isn't flexible bones but flexible brains. What I'm after is to restore each person to their human dignity.'[53]

There are two processes in working with Feldenkrais. Awareness Through Movement (ATM) sessions involve the therapist verbally guiding their client through a series of movements, drawing attention to how they move and encouraging them to use their attention, perception and imagination to discover more efficient and effective ways of moving.[53]

In Functional Integration (FI) sessions, the therapist moves the client, or uses their hands to guide the client's movement in patterns that will help restore awareness and balance.[53]

I commenced a series of Functional Integration sessions with a practitioner I had contacted through my work as a masseur. At each session, I lay supine on a low padded table while my practitioner moved quietly around me gently stretching or rearranging my limbs, pushing or just touching head, hands, face, hips. With each move, she tried to bring some balance back to my distorted, frail body while I entered a state close to trance and felt a 'connection' develop between my spirit, mind and body. I often felt quite euphoric as I left a session and had to be particularly careful while driving as it was easy to 'go off with the fairies' until I grounded myself again.

I enjoyed my FI sessions but the results were always temporary. Within a day or two, the sense of wellbeing and reduction in pain would dissipate and I would be back to square one. I was referred to Basil Glazer (a prominent Feldenkrais teacher) during his visit to Melbourne in 1996.

Basil's treatment was much stronger than my practitioner's.

He pulled and stretched my body in ways that seemed right and balancing at the time and, because of this, I did not object to the pain caused by the treatment. At the end of the session, I felt taller, stood straighter and moved with more assurance. I thought we had achieved a breakthrough. However, twenty-four hours later, I was in agonising pain. My whole body seemed to be cramping, aching and burning with deep, deep pain. My body had rebelled again. Some three days later, I was back in my pre-treatment state; very disappointed.

I decided not to pursue Feldenkrais as a therapy. This may have been a mistake. Had I persisted with my practitioner's treatment, I may well have made progress like 'Elizabeth' who recovered from Parkinson's disease using Feldenkrais as her form of bodywork.[54] However, I was short of money and tired of pain, so gave up.

My experience with all these bodywork modalities emphasises my view that *any and all bodywork for people with Parkinson's disease must be very gentle and nurturing.*

21

What is Trauma?
How Can I Repair the Effects?

The proposition that degenerative disorders may origi-
nate in unresolved stress or trauma during childhood is
supported by recent research showing long-term mental,
emotional and physical dysfunctions following childhood
stress of many types.[13,19]

As people with Parkinson's disease, we need to find ways
of understanding the circumstances that may have been
viewed by our body as traumatic, honouring that as part
of our growth to our current beauty, then finding ways of
resolving the initiating trigger.

During my work I have found many people who are not
aware of the initiating trauma, even though it seems obvious
to me, or who are not prepared to recognise the event or cir-
cumstance as traumatic. Sometimes the factors causing the
initial degeneration were seen as normal – eg. Father away at
war, systematic abuse common in the neighbourhood or at
school, an emotionally manipulative relationship with one
or both parents, inappropriate responsibility for siblings. In
these cases, we need to find a way to open emotional door-
ways and allow a change in the way our client views themselves
and their place in the world.

In some cases, the initiating trauma has occurred in the
womb. Where Mum is in an abusive relationship, or is close
to a person who dies suddenly, or suffers some other form of

trauma while pregnant, her stress hormones increase dramatically and can cross the placenta. Baby then becomes overloaded with cortisol, adrenaline and others during a critical time of growth and development.[13] This is nobody's fault; it just happens.

In fact, many of the initiating traumas are nobody's fault. We live in a world that presents us with many challenges. Some we deal with swiftly and surely, others we struggle with, and a few we cannot deal with at all.[13] That's life, so we may as well enjoy it while we can.

We can, however, change the way our body responds to traumatic events, even when they occurred long ago.

Many of you will already have sought help from counsellors of various types, hypnotherapists, kinesiologists and a wide range of energy and spiritual healing modalities. Some will find this concept entirely new and rather strange.

We don't yet understand the exact process of 'cell memory'. We do see, however, that childhood experiences impact on our physical health, mental health, ability to learn and our likelihood of developing chronic disorders.[13,19] We sense that this process, easily seen in stress physiology described earlier, affects us at a very deep level, perhaps even to our DNA.[13] In order to completely heal the initiating trauma, we must work at cell level, while continuing our journey with our emotions and spirit.

Two very useful therapies to help us are Medicine Tree's Trauma/Post Trauma homeopathic drops or spray, and flower essences.

Trauma/post trauma

This homeopathic complex contains eleven different remedies, some in a range of potencies. The combination is aimed at assisting resolution, at all levels, of traumatic events or circumstances. While it can be of benefit in treating recent traumas, I find it most useful in assisting the resolution of long past events. The action is often subtle and may not be noticed for some time. Some clients have told me that they are gaining no benefit from the remedy, while indicating unconsciously that the remedy is working.

For instance, one client had spent a year telling me that she was one of those people for whom the treatment would not work. She would like to get better, and would go on trying, but it wouldn't work. Three months after starting Trauma/Post Trauma, she was telling me how she gained no benefit from the remedy, while discussing her planned activities when she got well. My client had not noticed the change in language from 'it won't work' to 'when I get well'. Another client was very doubtful about the worth of the remedy, but explained that she had been experiencing 'moments of unexplainable joy' for the first time in her memory. Yet another client explained that he was experiencing 'happiness' for the first time in many years.

Trauma/Post Trauma seems to 'open the walls' we have built up around unbearably painful memories so we can process them with love and a minimum of pain. I have not had a client who is confronted with very painful or unmanageable issues. Rather, I find that opportunities arise to either explore past events and/or circumstances, or to refer my clients on to empathetic counsellors.

Trauma/Post Trauma is available in 10ml dropper bottles, or 20ml spray bottles. I usually find the spray bottles easier and they can be carried around and readily used by client or carer. Each spray is equivalent to approximately 2½ drops. I generally prescribe one spray twice daily for two weeks, then two sprays twice daily. I rarely find the need to prescribe more despite instructions on the bottle suggesting much higher doses.

155

Flower essences

These beautiful remedies may be used instead of Trauma/ Post Trauma or in conjunction with the homeopathic remedies as they work at different levels. I happen to use a combination of Bach Flower Remedies and Australian Bush Flower Essences, but there are many varieties of essences available and all work well when prescribed with love by a caring practitioner, or chosen by you, the person most knowledgeable about your needs. Find the range that resonates with you, and develop a way of selecting remedies that sit well with both you and your practitioner.

Flower Essences can be used to help resolve past trauma and/or to give support in the present. I often use my range of flower essences to help clients find a positive outlook in their current circumstances and focus of welcoming wellness. I use them myself to give support during change or challenging times.

It is often helpful to spend time with a skilled, empathetic counsellor discussing memories and feelings as you move toward wellness. You may find, as you use therapies such as the Aqua Hydration Formulas, Trauma/Post Trauma or Flower Essences, that your dreams change in character, or you develop different attitudes towards circumstances or people. You may even find memories of old experiences surfacing, allowing you to understand the impact they had on your life and changing your response to them.

Counsellors

Choosing a counsellor can be a little challenging as there are so many modalities offered, and descriptions of their work can be bewildering to those new to counselling. Perhaps the suggestions below will make the process a little easier.

1. Talk to your most trusted health practitioner about your desire for counselling and discuss the possibility of referral to a counsellor your practitioner knows and trusts.
2. When making a first appointment to see a counsellor, ask for a five-minute conversation on the telephone. You may find that you instantly 'feel at home' when talking to them, or that you don't want to see them after all. Trust your gut feeling. If the counsellor won't talk to you for five minutes, you probably don't want to see them.
3. Avoid counsellors of any modality who want you to commit to frequent sessions over a long period and/or want to prescribe drugs early in your relationship.
4. Talk to your friends and family to see if they have visited a counsellor, and whether they can recommend someone to you. You will be surprised at how many people you know who have gained benefit from counselling, and how empowering it is to ask for help.
5. If you see a counsellor, and you feel uncomfortable or feel that you are not 'getting anywhere', don't hesitate to change. On the other hand, if you feel comfortable with your counsellor, commit yourself to the process no matter how painful it might be from time to time.
6. My experience has been that a reasonable counselling process is to meet regularly for two or three months to deal with some important issues, then have a break for, say, three months before moving onto other issues. This gives you and your body time to assimilate all the new emotions expressed, and for your wallet to recover. A counsellor who helps you is worth whatever they charge, but sometimes we need a little break from the extra expense.
7. Keep your journal while you are seeing a counsellor. This will enhance the process.

Depression

One of the consequences of unresolved trauma from early life may be emotional challenges that are seen as, or diagnosed as, depression. Further, being diagnosed with Parkinson's disease, often by unsympathetic practitioners who give us no hope for taking any control over our lives,[21] may create or exacerbate feelings of depression or frustration.

Medical practitioners often see depression as one of the symptoms of Parkinson's disease.[21,45] It is assumed that most people with Parkinson's disease will suffer from depression at some stage of their disease process. In conservative therapy, this 'depression' is generally treated with anti-depressants, education about the conservative view of Parkinson's disease, and support from psychiatrists or similar therapists.[45]

Given the training, culture, network structure and diagnostic criteria of conservative practitioners, this seems to be both a reasonable diagnosis and appropriate treatment. In other words, good medicine.

But is it?

There is no doubt that you are likely to feel depressed from time to time. In fact, I would venture to say that everyone diagnosed with Parkinson's disease is depressed and frustrated at some time, whether you are ever diagnosed with clinical depression or not.

I would also venture to say that some individuals may display symptoms of clinical depression and need medication for a short to medium term. But I believe that you are unlikely to develop clinical depression unless this has been a challenge before diagnosis with Parkinson's disease.

Clinical depression is marked by a number of common symptoms:

- Mood change – despondency, despair, loss of interest in people, activities, sex and personal care.
- Sleep disturbance.
- Anorexia.
- Either suicidal tendencies or delusions.
- Difficulty in thought and concentration.
- Anxiety, irritability and/or aggression.
- Physical conditions such as fatigue, tiredness, loss of appetite, weight loss, constipation, bodily aches and pains, headaches, respiratory problems, dryness in the mouth and unusual sensations in chest or abdomen.
- A 'depressed' facial expression – frown, immobile face, down turned mouth, troubled expression.[1]

Your Parkinson's disease may cause you to exhibit some or most of these symptoms. In my experience to date, I have not seen a person diagnosed with Parkinson's disease who is truly anorexic or suicidal. However, all other symptoms in the above list are present to some degree in most of my patients at some time during their journey.

Does this mean you are depressed and require anti-depressant medication? I believe that this is very rare.

Parkinson's disease is frustrating, humiliating, imprisoning, and sometimes painful. Even before diagnosis, we are aware that we can no longer perform to our usual standard in areas of our daily life. As our disorder progresses, we lose energy, become clumsy, perhaps shake, find it difficult to walk, move, sit comfortably, sleep, and relate to our loved ones. We may have difficulty in eating, become constipated, lose our libido or suffer impotence. Some of us have to give up work and become dependent on others for our care.

Of course we become depressed!

We don't need drugs to suppress our feelings. We need

support, counselling, strategies and therapies that will give us a sense of worth, help us focus on the positive aspects of our life, and give us hope of something better.

It is important to remember that many anti-depressant drugs used today may exacerbate the symptoms of Parkinson's disease[1] (ask your health practitioner to read MIMS or a similar drug guide to fully understand how each drug may affect you). I often see clients who have been given anti-depressants for anxiety, find their tremor worsening, for instance, so have their levodopa medication increased, which increases dyskinesia, which in turn makes them more anxious because they feel they are getting worse.

Let's break the cycle.

How to help yourself if you feel depressed

There are a number of strategies and therapies that can help you move from a negative, hopeless, depressed state into a more positive and motivated emotional state.

1. **Keeping journals and notes.** Your weekly journal will help you understand that you really are making inroads against this debilitating disorder. Your practitioner's notes will give you extra information about your progress.

   Your spouse, carer, friends and family may like to keep their own notes on their observations, as these can often highlight tiny steps forward that can change our feelings about ourselves.

   Remember, progress will be slow and in small steps, so it is vital to keep your weekly journal.

2. **Setting goals.** Read the section on Goal Setting below and start to set goals regularly. Once you realise that you are really achieving something, your mood will change.

3. **Exercise.** Regular, rhythmic exercise like walking, swim-

ming, water aerobics, cross crawling, bike riding (even on an exercise bike) will help produce chemicals in the brain that give us feelings of pleasure. Discipline yourself to undertake regular exercise and, if possible, enlist the aid of a carer or family member to exercise with you. Even ten to fifteen minutes daily will help.

4. **Counselling**. It is often useful for a person with Parkinson's disease to talk to someone outside their daily circle about the issues that worry them. This may be your health practitioner, or someone trained in counselling – psychologist, psychotherapist, family counsellor or similar. Often just explaining your frustrations to someone who knows how to listen will relieve tension and lift depression. Hypnotherapy, Kinesiology or similar therapies may help you identify issues that are causing concern at a particular time, even if you are not fully aware of what they are.

5. **Flower Essence Therapy**. Flower essences are a subtle, yet powerful means of bringing a positive emotional change. Ask your health practitioner to support you with these lovely essences, or refer you to another practitioner skilled in flower essence therapy.

6. **Work with family and carers whenever possible.** Ask them to observe you and take note of any progress, however tiny. Ask them to talk about your progress whenever possible. The more encouraging remarks that are made, the more you will see how well you are doing.

7. **Use supplements or herbs**. There are a number of excellent dietary supplements and herbal combinations that can give you emotional support while dealing with issues of concern, without causing untoward side effects. Ask your health practitioner about these.

8. **Laugh**. Laughter is still 'the best medicine'. Laughter

releases endorphins and encephalins in our brain and helps us to 'feel good'. We can sometimes lift our gloom by generating laughter in even an artificial way. I often think about acting as drink waiter at a friend's wedding while I still had very severe Parkinsonian tremor; it always makes me laugh. I tell jokes, watch comedies on television, listen to radio commentators who make me laugh, associate with friends who are light-hearted. While ill, I learned to comment on funny happenings in my life, and laugh at my clumsiness. There is always something to laugh about, and who cares if nobody else thinks it's funny? Laughing is part of getting well, so indulge yourself with laughter every day.

In my experience, depression is usually a result of being trapped in a neurological disorder, rather than an internal symptom. You and your health practitioner can conquer this unwelcome visitor.

Healing past trauma is often best achieved with a combination of homeopathic remedies, Flower Essences, counselling and journaling. You are the person best able to judge the combination that suits you most, and this will probably change as time goes on. But be dedicated to the process; it is a critical part of your journey to wellness.

22

Setting Goals
and Living With Them

It's easy to say that our goal is to recover from Parkinson's disease. But we can't live with that goal, because everyone tells us it's impossible!

When I was almost incapacitated with Parkinson's disease in 1995, I could not face a goal of recovery. The task was too huge; I was too weak to walk to the front door or prepare a meal, so how could I recover?

I could, however, live with a goal of learning to walk to the front gate, or speaking three words without stammering, or preparing one simple meal each week.

Everyone who is diagnosed with Parkinson's disease thinks they want to recover. But you have probably been told that it is impossible. Anyway, you have probably never met anyone who has recovered, so it's really hard to believe that you can do it.

Talking about recovery is like talking about winning a major lottery, and it feels about as likely. It's a dream, but what we really want is to gain some energy, reduce our pain, stop shaking, be able to feed ourselves again and resolve our constipation.

You must also REALLY, REALLY want to get well and be prepared to work hard for a long time to achieve this. Breaking this long journey into smaller, more easily achievable steps will help you remain motivated and persistent.

So what sort of goals should you set? Obviously, the details depend on each individual. But, in general terms, you need to set goals that are achievable in a few weeks, are measurable objectively if possible, contribute to your health or lifestyle, and can lead to greater goals.

Examples:

- Drinking six glasses of pure water every day for two weeks.
- Walking 500 metres three times each week.
- Meditating for ten minutes each morning five days a week.
- Achieving the energy to cut the grass at home after two months.
- Starting back at lawn bowls after three month's treatment.
- Drinking from your drink bottle without aid.
- Lifting a spoon to your mouth once each day without spilling food.

As you can see, I am suggesting modest goals with a reasonable time limit. Even so, you may not achieve them within the given time. If this happens, it is important for you to have your journal, and be definite about the gains that have been made. Congratulate yourself on walking three hundred metres twice each week because you used not walk at all. Encourage yourself about the four glasses of water you are drinking on most days, and use that as incentive to achieve the full goal. And so on.

The examples of achievable goals I have given above are from actual cases. They were achieved; not always in the given time, but they *were* achieved. Other goals we have set at RETURN TO STILLNESS include doing 100 revolutions on an exercise bike each morning, walking to the front door without using a walking stick, tying shoe laces, fastening a belt, smiling, writing your name in less than five minutes.

The 'rules' for setting your goals are:

- Make sure the goal is achievable.
- Set goals for a few weeks or, at the most, a couple of months ahead. Two or three years is too far away.
- Make sure that you accept the goal and say out loud that you can (and will) achieve it.
- Talk about the goal and your progress towards it frequently with anyone who will listen, but do not criticise yourself if you are falling behind. Encourage yourself and congratulate yourself on progress so far.
- When one goal is achieved, set another.
- Whenever possible, involve your family and friends in setting goals so they can support you towards its achievement.
- **Keep a weekly journal.** This is the most important way to understand just how well you are doing, and how many goals you are achieving (see YOUR JOURNAL). Weekly notes on progress will help you see that you are making progress, and motivate you to strive a little harder.

Setting goals and living with them is a life skill important for all of us. It is extremely important for those attempting to achieve the 'impossible' – recovery from a neurological disorder.

23

Other Naturopathic Therapies

Herbal medicine

Western and Chinese herbal medicine have histories spanning thousands of years and, rightly, are held in high esteem by those who have experienced the great benefits of using herbs to enhance health. Many scientists and practitioners have worked to alleviate the symptoms of Parkinson's disease by using herbal medicines and have, indeed, brought comfort and support to many. However, there is little evidence that herbal medicine can actually reverse the degeneration creating Parkinson's disease symptoms.

My own experience leads me to the belief that herbal medicine is a wonderful adjunctive therapy to help us manage some of the more distressing symptoms while we use other therapies, as detailed earlier, to reverse the degenerative process. Digestive disturbances, constipation, blood pressure fluctuations, headaches, skin problems, fatigue, emotional challenges, infections, urinary disturbances and muscle weakness may all respond positively to appropriate herbal therapies.

In my view, it is important to seek guidance from a skilled naturopath or herbalist before embarking on herbal treatments. Herbs are powerful medicine, healing and strengthening when properly chosen and administered, but do pose certain, if mild, risks. Unwisely administered herbs may exacerbate symptoms, cause digestive problems or interact negatively with drug therapy or other complementary therapies.

Your skilled herbal practitioner will make a note of all other therapies you are using, explore your sensitivity to medicines and examine your daily routine, then choose herbs most likely to bring benefits without any adverse effects. When working with a herbalist, be sure to tell them about the dosage of homeopathics you take as this will give them a good idea about your sensitivity. I have found that herbs often work better when given in 'drop doses' rather than millilitres for those with Parkinson's disease. This is because of our innate sensitivity to all medicines and our underlying fragility. Often 6 to 20 drops of a herbal mix in a little water will have more benefit in chronic disease than 5 or 7 millilitres. Ask your herbalist to consider this when prescribing your remedy.

That being said, if you have developed a debilitating infection or another acute condition that requires rapid resolution, it may be necessary to prescribe the larger doses of herbs and observe your response closely.

If you are working with other practitioners, ask your herbalist to give you full details of the herbs prescribed so you can pass this on to your doctor and other therapists. This is really important. It is so easy for a caring and well-intentioned practitioner to prescribe a remedy that may interact with a herbal remedy unless they are kept up to date with what you are taking.

Despite my warning, do not hesitate to use herbal remedies to alleviate symptoms. They really work well. Herbs always taste a bit 'rugged', but their effect is worth that mild discomfort; and that can be reduced by taking the herbs in a little water or juice, or with food, unless your practitioner tells you otherwise.

Other modalities

We are blessed to live in countries where so many healing practices are allowed to flourish and are reasonably priced. Naturopathic and health-giving modalities come in a huge variety of guises, and research is adding to the range each year. Books and magazines explore and promote many new and newly discovered therapies or activities.

You have the right and responsibility to read about, ask about and research all you can. But keep your 'Shit Detector' at the ready. Many promoted therapies are based on theories that have a poor physiological grounding (and this is not restricted only to 'complementary' therapies; some Western medical theories are yet to be proven).

Where you feel a particular therapy or activity will be of benefit for you, talk to your primary health practitioners to make sure that there will be no clash with your current regime, then try it. You are the best judge of whether any particular therapy helps you or not.

Be cautious, but adventurous. There are many ways of getting well, and you may find the road that is just right for you.

24

Healing Modalities

Healing touch, spiritual healing and mind/body healing are the oldest forms of medicine we know. Before humans developed speech, they communicated love and care through touch, murmurs, other sounds, and a wide variety of gestures and actions indicating emotional support.

Today, there are so many practitioners offering healing in a myriad of forms that we can easily become confused and walk away from the great benefits healing modalities can bring.

We need to view the 'healing industry' with some caution. Many practitioners are simply offering Universal Healing Energy (God's healing, love healing, whatever you want to call it) that is available freely to all of us, at extraordinary prices that can only bring shame on themselves and the industry. On the other hand, there are practitioners who have developed wonderful skills in focusing healing energy and offer that to us at prices commensurate with the time involved and their need to maintain a modest lifestyle.

How do we tell the genuine practitioners from the 'quacks'? This is difficult because many 'quacks' appear to be respectable and skillful practitioners. It's easy to be cautious when self-proclaimed miracle healers tell us that they will 'cure' all our ills with a single touch, or that God works through them by performing miracles and if we give them lots of money, God will 'cure' us. However, we can be seduced by those who work more quietly and suggest we should see them weekly for many months (at very reasonable cost, of course), while they lay their hands on us and perform hypnotic rituals. Or, perhaps, they are Doctors of Integrative Medicine, flush with enthusiasm about mind/body medicine and asking us to trust them as they try out their newly learned Reiki rituals and push us to take huge quantities of vitamin pills.

Our best guide is our 'gut instinct'. Petrea King of Quest For Life in New South Wales[55] often talks about our 'Shit Detector', that little voice inside that says 'this is not right for me'. We need to listen to that voice. We also need to listen when the voice says 'this IS right for me'. There are many wonderful, genuine, loving practitioners of Reiki, Pranic Healing, Therapeutic Touch and many other forms of spiritual healing and healing touch who will bring comfort and support to your journey towards wellness.

The benefits received from genuine spiritual healing and healing touch are not, as often claimed, entirely imaginary or a placebo effect. There is sufficient scientific* evidence to convince all but the most obdurate objector that the benefits received from healing are not 'all in the mind'. In 'Placebo – Something for Nothing?' below, I allude to a double blind, randomised trial constructed to study the power of prayer.[56] Very significant benefits were noted in the 'prayed for group' as opposed to the 'not prayed for group'.[56]

---

*Scientific – The New Shorter Oxford English Dictionary lists three meanings of this word, all concerned with producing knowledge; *1. A person or institution concerned with science (especially natural science); 2. Based on the objective principles of scientific methodology; 3. Pertaining to Christian Science.* I am most concerned with the first definition, i.e. the pursuit of knowledge, while the science establishment seeks to limit the word to definition 2 which allows them to comfortably denigrate any new knowledge which does not fit within their arbitrarily imposed methodology. It is interesting to note that up to 80% of establishment drugs and therapies are yet to be fully proven efficacious and/or safe within the parameters of scientific methodology.

Some interesting research into hands-on healing (therapeutic touch) has been undertaken since the 1970's. The development of the Superconducting Quantum Interference Device (SQUID) has allowed the measurement of biomagnetic fields, including electromagnetic discharge from the hands of healers, while 1990's research has proven the benefits of Pulsed Electromagnetic Field therapy (PEMF) in enhancing the healing process following injury.[57]

Research over the last twenty years in a number of countries has shown that the hands of practicing healers emit biomagnetic waves which pulse between 0.2Hz and 20Hz, with the most intense concentration between 6Hz and 9Hz, which is precisely the range of electromagnetic waves used in PEMF therapy.[57]

PEMF therapy has been shown to result in:[57]

- enhanced capillary formation
- decreased necrosis
- reduced swelling
- pain reduction
- improved recovery of function
- skin wound reduction (in both depth and pain noted)
- reduction in muscle loss following ligament surgery
- improved tensile strength of ligaments
- acceleration of nerve regeneration.

It seems logical to assume that healers producing the same range of wavelengths will bring the same physical benefits.

Research from Israel has shown that practitioners can also produce radiant (infra-red) heat which increases cell growth, DNA, protein synthesis and cell respiration.[57]

A study on the 'Effects of Therapeutic Touch on Tension Headache Pain' was conducted by Keller and Bzdek in 1989.

Sixty volunteers with tension headaches were randomly divided into two groups. One group received five minutes of non-touching healing while the other group received the same attention but their 'therapists' concentrated on mental arithmetic during the session. There was a significant improvement in the condition of the 'healed' group, even allowing for the placebo response demonstrated by the placebo group.[57]

During my adventure with Parkinson's disease, I received healing many times in various forms including prayer, hands-on healing, absent healing and Reiki. Sometimes I was aware of an immediate response in my body (reduction in pain, improved mobility, enhanced sense of well-being), but often the healing activity blended into my general progress.

Another very interesting factor I noticed was that giving healing healed me. I was involved in both spiritual healing and healing in the form of Bowen Therapy and massage. I noticed that each time I gave healing or worked with a client, my symptoms improved. I was, and am, certain that I was not 'taking energy' from my clients. I could feel extra energy flow through me from 'the universe' to my client. When the healing or therapy was over and I closed my aura, it seemed that my 'energy tanks' had been refilled.

Many healers have told me that when they give healing or therapy, they also receive healing. Which leads me to the conclusion that, to paraphrase the Bible, it is just as blessed to give as it is to receive; and, when we receive healing from another, we give a gift of healing to them with no effort on our part.

All this means that there are a number of ways we can benefit from healing touch and spiritual healing. We can find a genuine practitioner who 'resonates' with us, whose work brings us a palpable feeling of comfort or strength, and who is willing to share our journey. We can also receive this same healing from all who love us if they are willing to look on us or touch us with deep, unconditional love. All loving touch is healing. All unconditional love is healing. Therefore, those who love us the most without condition are our most powerful healers.

As we begin the journey of loving ourselves without condition, we become our own healers, intimately involved in the process of restoring health to our body. At the same time, we become more able to give unconditional love to those around us, and benefit from the giving.

Placebo – something for nothing?

Placebo – *A pill, medicine, procedure, etc., prescribed more for the psychological benefit to the patient of being given a prescription than for any physiological effect. Also, a substance with no therapeutic effect used as a control in testing new drugs etc.; a blank sample in a test.* (The New Shorter Oxford English Dictionary).

Placebo – *a medicine that is ineffective but may help to relieve a condition because the patient has faith in its powers. New drugs are tested against placebos in clinical trials: the drug's effect is compared with the **placebo response**, which occurs even in the absence of any pharmacologically active substance in the placebo.* (Oxford Reference – Concise Medical Dictionary).

Placebo Effect – *A beneficial or adverse effect produced by a placebo which cannot be attributed to the placebo itself.* (The New Shorter Oxford English Dictionary).

A placebo, in terms of modern medical culture, is arbitrarily defined as a substance or therapy, the content of which is unable to be measured by Western scientific means. Within this context, therapies often defined as a placebo include homeopathy, flower essences, spiritual healing, prayer, Reiki, Bowen therapy, Craniosacral therapy, Feldenkrais, crystal healing, colour therapy, aura healing, and many other forms of 'energetic medicine'. Activities such as practitioner encouragement and positive feedback are also often ignored, considered unprofessional or written off as a placebo.

We must ask the question, however, does a true placebo exist? Western medicine seeks to prove the efficacy of its drugs by comparing the responses of patients receiving the drug with those receiving a placebo. However, in most cases, a significant percentage of the placebo patients show beneficial response even though they are receiving no recognised treatment.

One of the earliest documented placebo studies was conducted in 1799 at the Mineral Water Hospital by Dr. Haygarth and Dr. Falconer. They constructed a wooden replica of a device patented by Dr. Elisha Perkins of Connecticut that was claimed to be of benefit to those suffering from gout, rheumatism, headaches, epilepsy and other conditions.

Dr. Haygarth tested the placebo device with five patients on the 6th January 1799. All claimed at least some improvement from the treatment with some being significantly better. The patients were later treated with Dr. Perkins' patented device with almost identical results.[58]

True 'scientific' studies are 'double blind, randomised and placebo controlled'. This means that neither the patient nor their doctor knows whether the drug or placebo is being supplied, and patients within the group being studied (the 'population') are selected at random by the authors of the study to receive the drug or placebo in order to eliminate bias.

So how can an inert, non-therapeutic substance bring a beneficial response? Further, if a placebo brings health improvement to a large number of people (which scientists tell us it does), is it ethical or, indeed, obligatory to make use of the placebo response in treating illness?

Elwyn Rees, a scientist with extensive qualifications and wide experience in a number of scientific disciplines, believes that a placebo does not actually exist because it is incapable of definition in strict scientific terms.[59] Rees argues persuasively that definition of a placebo to date ignores factors such as psychology, feedback, time and space matrix and bio-energetic challenge. In speaking of 'placeboists' (those who seek to define 'placebo') he says, 'Lacking scientific definitions and the stringent criteria analysis demanded by comprehensive, wide-band, time-space monitoring regimes crucial to bio-energetic research, his contribution begins to risk appearing, at best, unscientific and, at worst, dangerous'.[59]

While Rees's views are refreshing in causing us to rethink the place placeboes may play in our own practice, 'placebo' is a useful umbrella term to cover those therapies and activities so long neglected by the scientific/medical community because they are 'useless, dangerous, unethical' or simply not understood except as a vehicle to 'prove' that drugs are effective.

Ernst and Abbot believe that most clinicians will not recognise a placebo effect because their experience has not encompassed the administration of a pure placebo, they are unwilling to withhold recognised therapy in favour of a placebo (believing it to be unethical) and have no means of judging (nor any desire to judge) how much of the beneficial effect arising from any given therapy may, in fact, be a placebo response.[58]

The benefit of understanding a placebo and its possibilities is that it comes free with every therapy given.[58] If the therapy is administered by a caring, positive practitioner, then a placebo is positively good. If the administration or practitioner is negative or uncaring, then the placebo effect is likely to be negative.

An anecdotal example comes from my own experience (and there are many who can relate similar experiences). My neurologist told me, 'When you get worse . . .' ; in other words, he was saying that degeneration was inevitable and I had no hope of reversing the process. I felt an immediate sense of hopelessness and fear for the future.

On the other hand, my craniosacral therapist asked me what I wanted to do about my condition, and joined with me to make a plan for recovery. With these words, she gave me back the power to control my life and continue to search, with hope, for a pathway to health.

I believe that health professionals have an obligation to give our clients the power of hope and positive thought, knowing that a significant number will respond well to this even if the words are 'placebo'.

However, we do not have to rely on anecdotes to see the healing power of 'placebo'.

Randolph Byrd, a cardiologist in California, conducted a ten-month randomised, prospective, double blind study on prayer. Three hundred and ninety-three coronary patients receiving standard medical care were computer assigned to a 'prayed for group' or a 'non-prayed for group'. Those prayed for were five times less likely to require antibiotics, three times less likely to develop pulmonary oedema, none required mechanical respiration and mortality was significantly lower than in the non-prayed for group.[56]

The prayed for group did not know they were receiving this 'therapy' yet responded well. Can we, therefore, conclude that prayer, and its counterparts such as spiritual healing, is a valid therapy worthy of greater study? In medical terms, certainly. In the terms of non-medical therapists, we've known it all along and should pursue this avenue vigorously whenever possible.

Kai Kermani, a medical doctor and psychic healer, relates three cases of patients suffering intractable pain who recovered when given absent healing.[60] The many stories such as this in clinical files throughout the world, plus the many stories of 'spontaneous remissions' and 'unexplainable miracles' which abound, serve to reinforce the view that spiritual healing in its many forms is positive healing energy and a valid health therapy.

Ernst and Abbot say 'So we can't disregard or downgrade the placebo effect: it is a part of the bloom of therapeutic improvement as surely as petals are part of a flower'.[58]

While the physiological actions of 'energetic therapies' such as homeopathy, flower essences, spiritual healing, prayer, Reiki, Bowen therapy, Craniosacral therapy, Feldenkrais, crystal healing, colour therapy, aura healing and positive encouragement require study and explanation when we are able to find appropriate measurement techniques, we can safely accept that they work to the positive benefit of the recipients and that a placebo is 'something for nothing'.

When choosing your therapist, or the company you keep, remember that the 'placebo effect' is present in every word we hear or touch we receive. Choose wisely and respect your healing journey. In my view, 'placebo' is the most powerful medicine in the world, and it's free!

25

Carers

A letter to Carers

Dear Carer,
You are a vital key to recovery. You can enhance the road or act as an almost impenetrable barrier.

You may be a spouse, child, sibling, friend or employee. You may be the instigator of your loved one's first contact with the practitioner who diagnosed Parkinson's disease, the person who bought this book for your loved one, an unconvinced observer, or highly resistant to spending money on anything other than conservative Western therapy.

You have a very hard road as you watch your loved one degenerate or struggle to recover. Many of you speak tearfully to me about the 'person you used to know' – active, bright, loving – and how they have deteriorated into a dependent, remote, humiliated person. Yet some of you are unwilling to move out of conservative care, even though your loved one may be desperate to try anything that gives hope of even a marginal improvement in health.

When you decide to support recovery, you provide a wonderful resource to assist your loved one on their journey. Help as much as you can without imposing burdens on yourself.

You can observe your loved one and often see changes that they are not aware of. You can keep your own journal or write your observations in your loved one's journal. Your information is extremely valuable.

You can be 'medicine managers', reminding your loved one about their various pills and drops at the right time.

You can encourage, support, cajole, persuade and congratulate. I find that a team of three can be at least twice as effective as a team of two, so become involved in visits to practitioners, goal setting and all other activities on the journey.

You can make all the difference. You are a wonderful resource for healing.

John Coleman, ND

If you don't have a carer who supports you

During my recovery process, there was no one person by my side. My regular visits to various practitioners became visits to 'family', because these were the people who knew me best and observed changes most perceptively. Without their encouragement and stabilising influence, I doubt that I could have recovered. Perhaps this will happen for you too if you do not have a specific carer by your side.

Be very open and honest with your practitioners. Tell them how you feel physically and emotionally. If you find them reluctant to listen, find another practitioner.

Relationship difficulties frequently occur when one partner develops a serious illness. Often these difficulties can be overcome with patience and conversation, especially if there is great love between you. There may be occasion where it is beneficial for you both to see an appropriate counsellor or other therapist to deal with specific issues.

Where you find that your carer is resistant to some activity that you see as important for your recovery, sit down and talk to them quietly and with love. It is so difficult to understand how you feel inside without your experience. All your carer can see is what is on the outside. All they can understand is what you tell them. So be very open and patient in explaining what you are feeling, what you want to do, why it will cost time and/or money, and how they can be a vital part of your progress.

If you feel you have no support, ask your practitioner about linking up with others on this same journey. Perhaps you can help each other. Join groups such as the Neuro Recovery Foundation, meditation classes and discussion groups. There are often people willing to listen to your concerns, and support you along the way.

26

Frequently Asked Questions

Have you found a cure for Parkinson's disease?

No. there is still no 'cure' known for Parkinson's disease. The word 'cure' implies that you want someone to give you a drug, herb, vitamin or operation that will take away all your symptoms and stop them returning. That just can't happen. However, you can RECOVER. This means that you can harness all your own resources, and work with practitioners, family and friends to reverse the degenerative processes that led to the symptoms of Parkinson's disease.

Do I have to stop taking my drugs to recover?

No. It is important to continue taking any drugs prescribed by your doctor while you begin your journey of recovery. Many drugs are useful in giving comfort and support while you work slowly to regain balance in your body. Over a long time, you can work with your practitioners to very slowly reduce your drug intake as and when your body shows that you are ready to do that.

Will any of the therapies suggested in this book conflict with medicine prescribed by my doctor?

In general, the answer is no. However, there are a few examples of herbs interacting with drugs, so you need to consult a skilled practitioner before taking herbal remedies.

No homeopathic or flower essence remedies will conflict in any way with drug therapy. Please make sure you let each practitioner know exactly what you are taking so that each can make appropriate choices of therapy to give you the best possible progress toward health.

How long will it take for me to get well?

The simple answer is 'as long as it takes'. Each person is different, with individual backgrounds, experiences, genetic make up, attitudes, environments and beliefs. Every factor of our life affects our health, including belief and attitude. So your journey to health will take as long as it takes you to make the changes in and around you necessary to find wellness. For some, that is three or four years; for others, perhaps five or six years. There will be many changes and achievements along the way, and every moment of our journey is important. Getting well requires patience, dedication, love and, most of all, the knowledge that every experience is an opportunity to learn and grow, and become healthier in the truest sense.

Will I get worse before I get better?

No. But sometimes you will think you're getting worse. Our progress to health fluctuates according to what is happening in and around us on any given day. Sometimes we feel we have been making progress for a while, then we suffer a setback for some reason; our symptoms seem to get worse again and we feel we are slipping back. There is always a reason this happens – perhaps we are developing an infection, or there are some problems in the family, work has become more stressful, or perhaps we are at the stage of needing to make a small adjustment to our medication. Talk honestly to your health practitioner about how you are feeling, and look back at your journal to understand how recent events may be affecting you. You are not 'getting worse again', but you are learning something important about your health.

Will I need to take the same remedies all the time?

Probably not. As your health status changes, you may find it necessary to review your drug and remedy regime. Make regular contact with your health practitioners and keep a note of symptoms in your journal. My experience indicates that you will need the Aqua Hydration Formulas for a long time, plus a fluctuating regime of homeopathics, supplements, possibly herbs, plus sensible use of Western medication.

Do I need to tell my doctor what I'm doing?

I believe it is important to be open with all your health practitioners. It is very difficult for doctors, naturopaths, homeopaths and herbalists to give the best care if we don't know what medicines or other therapies you have chosen to use. There is a small possibility of interaction between therapies but, more importantly, we need to understand what is helping you and what is hindering your progress. So please tell your doctor that you are taking homeopathics, supplements, etc., and leave a list of remedies with them. Your doctor may not be interested in any other therapy, of course, but should be informed of your choices. If you are unfortunate enough to attend a doctor who becomes angry or aggressive when you tell them about your choices (and some do), I suggest you look for another doctor.

Can my doctor forbid me to make choices about my health?

No. Your doctor is skilled in one important form of medicine and, in general, will do his or her best to give you the optimum treatment for your individual needs and disorder. However, you are free to discuss treatments with your doctor, suggest modifications or compromises, and undertake any other form of therapeutic activity that is right for you. Your doctor has every right to express an opinion about your choices, but cannot dictate to you what you may or may not do.

If I have other health challenges such as high blood pressure, arthritis, diabetes or heart disease as well as Parkinson's disease, can I still use the remedies suggested in this book?

In general, the therapies suggested will be of assistance in alleviating other health challenges too. However, you need to discuss your individual needs with each of your health practitioners and make choices about the best regime just for you. I have worked with people with Parkinson's disease who also display many other health challenges and, in each case, we have seen their overall health improve as their Parkinson's disease symptoms diminish. Be very open with your health practitioners to ensure you are getting the best possible treatment for you as a complete and perfect person.

How will I know when I'm well?

When you wake up each morning looking forward to the day ahead, feeling plenty of energy to undertake the tasks you have chosen, and knowing you are happy with the company you have chosen, then you are well. Congratulations!

27

Is That all There is?

It seems so complicated, doesn't it? There are things to do, people to see, dietary changes, therapies you've never heard of, stuff that seems a bit weird.

It's really quite simple.

Your journey to health begins the moment you make up your mind to make a change. Any change, no matter how small.

You are the only person who can make healthy changes, and the time to do it is NOW. Don't wait until your next visit to your neurologist, or after you've talked to the children who are all a bit busy at the moment, or after you've paid off the DVD player, or when you've finished this bottle of Sinemet, or when you have more energy.

No matter how advanced your Parkinson's disease, you can make healthy choices, and change your life NOW.

Go through this book again and highlight all the bits that resonate with you. Put 'Stick On Notes' on those pages, or turn down the corners (I won't object, I promise) so you can refer to them quickly whenever you want to. Then set off on this wonderful journey, step by step.

1. Know that you have a real desire to be as healthy as you possibly can be.
2. Acknowledge that it is YOUR responsibility to change your state of health.
3. Acknowledge and honour your past, whatever that may

be, as the path by which you reached this point of understanding and challenge.

4. Understand that the past cannot be changed and is not your fault. 'Shit happens'.
5. Look in the mirror and say 'I love you'.
6. Gather around you those who love you without condition or expectation, and whom you love unconditionally. Walk away from those who want you for what you do.
7. Understand that YOU are the 'expert' on your health and work only with those who honour that.
8. Keep a Journal.
9. Review your diet.
10. De-toxify your life.
11. Laugh, relax, meditate. Be happy NOW.
12. Hydrate your cells.
13. Deal with the initiating trauma using Homeopathics, Flower Essences, Counselling, Kinesiology and/or other ways that suit you.
14. Use Bowen Therapy and other bodywork to give you comfort and enhance your progress towards wellness.
15. Have a great adventure!

Parkinson's disease is your challenge and your privilege. You can give up now and descend into an expected state of humiliating degeneration, or you can take control, accept your responsibility and begin your journey to wellness.

Your state of health is up to YOU.

You CAN get well.

Useful Websites and Other Resources

<www.neurorecoveryfoundation.com.au> the neuro recovery foundation was founded in 2002 to enhance the distribution of information about all neurological disorders to those diagnosed, family and friends. The foundation seeks to find and disseminate information about recovery and supportive therapies, while supporting the rational use of Western medicine. Phone 0500 512 000 for brochures.

<www.questforlife.com.au> established by Petrea King many years ago, the Quest For Life Foundation and Centre in Bundanoon, New South Wales, provides many wonderful residential programmes for those with chronic, debilitating illnesses, and those wishing to enhance their life. Programmes include Neuro Recovery Pathways for those diagnosed with neurological disorders.

<www.returntostillness.com.au> this is my own website and includes some of my story, plus case histories. Contact details are included.

<www.hydration.org> the official website of Wild Medicine, manufacturers of the Aqua Hydration Formulas with details of their contents, development and directors of the company.

'Returning To Stillness': a small booklet telling my story of illness and recovery sold through the neuro recovery foundation inc. The cost is $20 with profits going to the foundation.

'Elizabeth's Story': another small booklet telling the story of Elizabeth who recovered from Parkinson's disease some years ago. Again, you can obtain this through the neuro recovery foundation inc. with proceeds supporting the work of the foundation.

Neuro Recovery Pathways: residential programmes for those challenged with any neurological disorder, conducted at the Quest For Life Centre in NSW several times each year. Check details on the Quest For Life website, or call 02 4883 6599.

<www.feldenkrais-resources.com> extensive information about Feldenkrais.

<www.craniosacral.com> lots of information about Craniosacral Therapy.

References

1. *MIMS Annual 2004*: published MIMS Australia, St. Leonards, NSW, Australia.
2. *The Mosby Medical Encyclopedia* (Revised Edition); Plume; Penguin Books, Ringwood, Victoria, Australia, 1992.
3. Larsen J.P., Dupont E., Tandberg E.; 'Clinical diagnosis of Parkinson's disease. Proposal of diagnostic subgroups classified at different levels of confidence'; *ACTA Neurologica* Scandanavia 1994: 89; pp 242–51.
4. *Oxford Textbook of Medicine*, third edition; Oxford University Press, 1996; Volume 3, Section 24.10; pp 3998–4005.
5. *The MERCK Manual*, fourteenth edition; 1982; pp 1357–62, 2335, 2337.
6. Montgomery Erwin B. Jr.; 'Heavy metals and the etiology of Parkinson's disease and other movement disorders'; *Toxicology* 97 (1995); pp 3–9.
7. Lewy Body Pathology; Tripod Website; http://sabryabdelfattah. tripod.com/docs/LEWY.htm; downloaded 26th March 2005.
8. McCance Kathryn L., Huether Sue E.; *Pathophysiology – The Biologic Basis for Disease in Adults and Children*; The C.V. Mosby Company, 1990; pp 445, 454, 455, 509–13.
9. 'Extrapyramidal Syndromes of Abnormal Posture or Involuntary Movement'; *Degenerative Diseases of the Nervous System*; Chapter 373; pp 1997–99.
10. Marsden C.D., Obeso J.A.; 'The functions of the basal ganglia and the paradox of stereotaxic surgery in Parkinson's disease'; *Brain* (1994), 117; pp 877–97.
11. Starr Michael S.; 'Glutamate/Dopamine D_1/D_2 Balance in the Basal Ganglia and Its Relevance to Parkinson's disease'; *Synapse* 19 (1995); pp 264–93.
12. Iansek Robert; 'Parkinson's disease; practical approach to treatment'; *Current Therapeutics*, October 1995; pp 55–60.

13. Victoroff Dr. Jeff; *Saving Your Brain;* Bantam Books (Random House Australia), Milsons Point, NSW, Australia, 2002.
14. *Medicines: The Comprehensive Guide*; The Book Creation Company, U.K., 1991.
15. Larsen Hans R.; 'Parkinson's – victory in sight?'; *International Journal of Alternative and Complementary Medicine*, Vol 15 No. 10, October 1997; pp 22–4.
16. Daniel Jacqueline R., Mauro Vincent F.; 'Extrapyramidal Symptoms Associated with Calcium-channel Blockers'; *The Annals of Pharmacotherapy*, Volume 29, January 1995; pp 73–5.
17. *Parkinson's Australia Magazine*, Winter 1998, Number 9.
18. Bernstein Ken; 'Evaluating Disease Severity'; excerpted from *Parkinson's Disease Handbook*, American Parkinson's Disease Association (APDA); downloaded from Parkinson's Web (internet) 1998.
19. McEwen Professor Bruce; interview by Dr. Norman Swan on ABC Radio National 'The Health Report' 10th January 2005; downloaded from ABC website 11th January 2005.
20. 'Parkinson's Disease'; *The Physician's Handbook of Clinical Nutrition*, Chapter 12, Nutritional Physiology of the Brain; pp 262–4 (excerpt provided by Bio Concepts, Queensland, Australia).
21. Marjama-Lyons Jill, M.D.; *What Your Doctor May Not Tell You About Parkinson's Disease*; Warner Books, New York, USA; 2003.
22. Swank Roy Laver, M.D., Ph.D. & Dugan Barbara Brewer; *The Multiple Sclerosis Diet Book*; Doubleday, New York, USA; 1987.
23. JelinekProfessor George, M.D.; *Taking Control of Multiple Sclerosis*; Hyland House Publishing, Flemington, Victoria, Australia; 2000.
24. Croxson S., Johnson B., Millac P., Pye I.; 'Dietary modification of Parkinson's disease'; *European Journal of Clinical Nutrition* (1991), 45; pp 263–6.
25. Briggs David, Wahlqvist Mark; *Food Facts*; Penguin Books Australia Ltd; 1988.
26. Burk-Shull Kathleen A.; 'Protein redistribution to improve quality of life for those with Parkinson's disease: A review'; *Topics in Clinical Nutrition* 1994; 10(1); pp 65–70.
27. Berry E.M., Growdon J.H., Wurtman J.J., Caballero B., Wurtman R.J., 'A balanced carbohydrate:protein diet in the management of Parkinson's disease'; *Neurology* 1991; 41; pp 1295–7.

References

28. Giminez-Roldan S., Mateo D.; 'Predicting beneficial response to a protein-redistribution diet in fluctuating Parkinson's disease'; *Acta neurology*, Belgium, Vol 91, 1991; pp 189–200.
29. Oyston Eleanor; 'A Simple Explanation of the Science of Bowen Therapy'; unpublished; 2004.
30. Boublik Dr. Jaroslav; 'The Hydration Equation'; *Diversity Natural and Complementary Health* Volume 2 No 3, Sept–Nov 2000; pub Australian Complementary Health Association, Melbourne Australia.
31. Abrahams Professor Peter; *The Atlas of the Human Body*; Thunder Bay Press, California, USA; 2002.
32. <www.hydration.org>; official website for Wild Medicine, manufacturers of the Aqua Hydration Formulas.
33. 'Homeopathic Medicine Potency or Dilution'; no author given; <www.ritecare.com/homeopathic/guide-potency.asp>; downloaded from website 25th March 2005.
34. Chaltin Luc, N.D., D.I., Hom.; 'Understanding Homeopathy – Homeopathic Potencies or Attenuations'; <www.pets4homeopathy.com>; downloaded 25th March 2005.
35. Kotok Alexander, M.D.; 'The History of Homeopathy in the Russian Empire Until World War I as compared with Other European Countries and the USA: similarities and discrepancies'; PhD thesis, 2001.
36. Coulter Catherine R.; *Portraits of Homeopathic Medicines*; North Atlantic Books; Berkeley, California, USA; 1986.
37. Callinan Paul; *Australian Family Homeopathy*; Viking/Penguin Books Australia Ltd; Ringwood, Victoria, Australia; 1995.
38. Kabat-Zinn Jon, Ph.D.; *Full Catastrophe Living*; Delta Book; Dell Publishing, New York, USA; 1990.
39. 'Meditation'; no author given; <www.wholehealthmd.com>; downloaded from website 16th January 2005.
40. Large Elizabeth; 'Meditation finally gets credit for health benefits'; *Island Life*; <www.honoluluadvertiser.com>; downloaded from website 16th January 2005.
41. Flanagan Dr. Gael Crystal and Dr. Patrick; 'Laughter – Still the Best Medicine'; <www.heylady.com/rbc/laughter.htm>; downloaded 25th January 2005.
42. Doskoch Peter; 'Happily Ever Laughter'; *Psychology Today*: July/August 1996.

43. Welch Susan; 'The Best Medicine'; *Sunday Herald Sun*, January 30, 2005, Melbourne, Australia.
44. Borge Victor; 'Quotations By Subject'; *The Quotations Page*; <www.quotationspage.com>; downloaded 30th January 2005.
45. Oxtoby Dr. Marie, Williams Professor Adrian, with Iansek Professor Robert; *Parkinson's At Your Fingertips*; The McGraw-Hill Companies, Inc. Sydney, Australia, 2002.
46. Coleman John, N.D.; *Returning To Stillness*; self published; available through the neuro recovery foundation inc. <www.neurorecovery-foundation.com.au>.
47. Baker Julian; 'Less is more'; *International Journal of Alternative and Complementary Medicine*, Vol 14 No 12, December 1996; pp 16–18.
48. Stammers Glen; 'The Bowen Technique'; *WellBeing Magazine*, International Edition, No 65; pp 88–9.
49. Morling Greg; 'Parkinson's disease and massage therapy'; *International Journal of Alternative and Complemenatry Medicine*, Vol 16 No 3, March 1998; pp 24–5.
50. Chaitow Leon; 'Energy and bodywork'; *International Journal of Alternative and Complementary Medicine*, Vol 15 No 8, August 1997; pp 28–32.
51. Chaitow Leon; 'Muscular influences on cranial dysfunction'; *International Journal of Alternative and Complementary Medicine*, Vol 16 No 1, January 1998; pp 30–2.
52. Chaitow Leon; 'Muscular influences on cranial dysfunction'; *International Journal of Alternative and Complementary Medicine* Vol 16 No 2, February 1998; pp 31–3.
53. 'Feldenkrais'; a training brochure produced by the Australian Feldenkrais Guild Inc.
54. 'Elizabeth's Story'; published by the neuro recovery foundation inc.
55. <www.questforlife.com.au>; official website of the Quest For Life Foundation and Centre.
56. Callinan Paul; 'Miracles in Medicine'; *WellBeing Magazine*, International Edition, Number 65; pp 12–16.
57. Chaitow Leon; 'Energy and bodywork'; *International Journal of Alternative and Complementary Medicine*, Vol 15 No 6, June 1997; pp 31–3.

References

58. Ernst Professor Edzard, Abbot N.C.; 'Uncovering the placebo in disguise'; *International Journal of Alternative and Complementary Medicine*, Vol 16 No 4, April 1998; pp 11–12.
59. Rees Elwyn; 'Why placebo does not please'; *International Journal of Alternative and Complementary Medicine*, Vol 16 No 8, August 1998; pp 18–23.
60. Kermani Kai; 'Healing past-life wounds'; *International Journal of Alternative and Complementary Medicine*, Vol 16 No 8, August 1998; pp 15–17.

Glossary of Terms

Acetylcholine: a neurotransmitter that enables muscles to contract.[2]

Acupuncture: an ancient Eastern therapy in which fine needles are inserted into the skin at specific points along a series of lines called meridians. The needles may be twirled, given a slight electric charge or warmed.[2]

Akinesia: an abnormal state of mental and physical inactivity or inability to move the muscles.[2]

Anorexia: a loss of appetite that results in the person not being able to eat.[2] It is a serious condition that may result in illness or death.

Aspartame: a white, almost odourless crystalline powder with an intensely sweet taste. It is used as an artificial sweetener. It is about 180 times as sweet as the same amount of sugar.[2] Aspartame is very neurotoxic.

Ataxia: a blocked ability to coordinate movements.[2]

Autonomic: having the ability to function independently without outside influence; eg. the autonomic nervous system.[2]

Basal ganglia: the islands of grey matter within each one of the lobes of the brain (cerebrum). They are involved in posture and coordination.[2]

Benserazide: a dopa decarboxylase inhibitor contained in Madopar to reduce the amount of levodopa absorbed into tissue, thus increasing the amount of levodopa available across the blood brain barrier.

Bilateral: occurring on both sides of the body.

Bioindividuality: our uniqueness as individuals.

Bradykinesia: an abnormal condition characterised by slowness of all bodily movement and speech.[2]

Carbidopa: a dopa decarboxylase inhibitor contained in many levodopa drugs to reduce the amount of levodopa absorbed into tissue, thus increasing the amount of levodopa available across the blood brain barrier.

Caudate nucleus: part of the basal ganglia, concerned with movement.[31]

Cerebrospinal fluid: the fluid that flows through and protects the brain and spinal canal.[2]

Glossary of Terms

Chiropractic: a system of body therapy based on manipulations of the spine.[2]

Complemenatry Medicine: systems of medicine that fall outside the purview of conservative Western medicine. Often called Natural Medicine or Alternative Medicine.

Complementary Therapies: therapies practiced under the umbrella of Complementary Medicine.

Craniosacral Therapy: a gentle, hands-on method of evaluating and enhancing the functioning of a physiological body system called the craniosacral system – comprised of the membranes and cerebrospinal fluid that surround and protect the brain and spinal cord.

Cupping: a technique of applying a suction device ('cup') to the skin to draw blood to the surface of the body.[2]

Cure: medical treatment; curing or preserving fish, pork, etc; the process of curing rubber or plastic. (ref: *The New Shorter Oxford Dictionary,* 1993)

Decarboxylase inhibitor: a drug added to levodopa preparations to reduce the amount of levodopa absorbed into tissue before crossing the blood brain barrier.

Dopamine: a neurotransmitter normally produced in the brain. It may be deficient in those displaying the symptoms of Parkinson's disease.

Dyskinesia: impaired ability to make voluntary movements and/or unusual and abnormal movements caused by disease or drug therapy.[2]

Dysphagia: difficulty in swallowing.[2]

Dyspnea: shortness of breath or difficulty in breathing.[2]

Efficacy: the greatest ability of a drug or treatment to produce a result, regardless of dosage.[2]

Endorphin: substances composed of amino acids, produced by the pituitary gland and acting on the nervous system to reduce pain. They produce effects like morphine.[2]

Epidemiology: the study of the spread, prevention and control of disease in a community or group of persons.[2]

Feldenkrais: a bodywork modality developed by Moshe Feldenkrais to facilitate the 'integration of the skeletal, developmental, environmental and neuromuscular systems'.[53] It offers a framework in which the patterns of movement, thought and feeling can be explored.[53]

Festinating: a way of walking in which the person increases speed in an unconscious effort to 'catch up' with a displaced centre of gravity.[2]

Free radical: an unstable compound that reacts quickly with other molecules.[2]

Gamma interferon: a natural protein found in cells when they are exposed to a virus or other foreign materials. It stimulates production of a protein in neighbouring cells that stops the growth of the virus, thus protecting them from infection.[2]

Gliosis: reparative or pathological proliferation of glial cells (in the brain). (ref: *The New Shorter Oxford Dictionary*, 1993)

Homeopath: a practitioner specialising in homeopathy.

Homeopathy: a system of healing based on the theory of 'like cures like'; developed by Dr. Samuel Hahnemann in the late 18th century; using very small doses.[2]

Homocysteine: an amino acid in the blood. Epidemiological studies have shown that too much homocysteine in the blood (plasma) is related to a higher risk of coronary heart disease, stroke and peripheral vascular disease. (ref: <www.americanheart.org>)

Hypertension: a common disorder, often without symptoms, marked by high blood pressure persistently exceeding 140/90.[2]

Hypertonic: long-term muscle contracture as a result of constant nerve stimulation.[2]

Hypnotherapy: the use of hypnosis along with other techniques in psychotherapy.[2]

Hypotension: an abnormal condition in which the blood pressure is too low for normal functioning.[2]

Hypothalamus: a portion of the brain, forming the floor and part of the side wall of the third ventricle. It activates, controls and integrates part of the nervous system, the endocrine processes, and many bodily functions, such as temperature, sleep and appetite.[2]

Hypotonic: long-term muscle relaxation as a result of poor nerve message transmission.

Idiopathic: without a known cause.[2]

Immunoglobulin: any of five structurally and antigenically distinct antibodies in the serum and external secretions of the body. In response to certain antigens, immunoglobulins are formed in the bone marrow, spleen and all lymphoid tissue of the body except the thymus.[2] Part of our immune response.

Impotence: inability of the adult male to achieve erection or, less commonly, to ejaculate having achieved an erection.[2]

Interaction: the way medicines of various types might enhance or inhibit the actions of each other.

Levodopa: a chemical precursor to dopamine. May be created in the body or taken as a drug.

Lewy bodies: clumps of protein found in the cytoplasm of certain brain cells, typically in people with Parkinson's disease.[21]

Libido: the psychic energy or instinctual drive associated with sexual desire, pleasure, or creativity.[2]

Locus caeruleus: a specific part of the basal ganglia in the brain.

Lymph: a thin, clear, slightly yellow fluid originating in many organs and tissues of the body.[2] Part of our drainage and immune systems.

Metaphysical: transcends matter or the physical. (ref: *The New Shorter Oxford Dictionary*, 1993)

MRI (magnetic resonance imaging): an imaging technique used in medicine that employs nuclear magnetic resonance of protons in the body. (ref: *The New Shorter Oxford Dictionary*, 1993)

Multi System Atrophy: a progressive, degenerative disorder of the brain, similar to Parkinson's disease, affecting many bodily functions.

Naturopath: a practitioner employing naturopathic techniques to assist patients recover.

Naturopathy: a system of disease treatment using natural foods, light, warmth, massage, fresh air, regular exercise, and the avoidance of drugs. Supporters believe that illness can be healed naturally by the body.[2]

Necrosis: local tissue death that occurs in groups of cells because of disease or injury.[2]

Neuroendocrine: pertaining to or involving both nervous stimulation and endocrine secretion. (ref: *The New Shorter Oxford Dictionary*, 1993)

Neuroprotective: substances or activities that may protect nerve cells or the nervous system.

Neurotoxic: substances or activities that may damage nerve cells or the nervous system.

Neurotransmitter: any chemical that changes or results in the sending of nerve signals across spaces (synapses) separating nerve fibres.[2]

Nocturnal Micturition: urination during the night.

Omega 3 fatty acids: a group of essential fatty acids (ie. must be obtained from food) prevalent in flax seed oil, fish, avocado and similar foods, required for cell health, appropriate cholesterol levels and general health.

Pathophysiology: development of a disease state.

Procyanidin: the active antioxidant element in various foods such as grape seeds.

Putamen: part of the basal ganglia that receives input from the cerebral cortex.[31]

Recover: restore to health, strength or consciousness; regain health, strength or consciousness after; get better from. (ref: *The New Shorter Oxford Dictionary*, 1993)

Reflux: an abnormal backward or return flow of a fluid, as when stomach contents go back into the gullet (esophagus) to cause heartburn.[2]

Reiki: a philosophy of spiritual healing involving specific teaching and rituals.

Sensitivity: the quality or degree of being sensitive or responsive – eg. to medicine or environment.

Substantia nigra: a curved layer of grey matter on each side of the mid brain, separating the tegmentum from the crus cerebri. (ref: *The New Shorter Oxford Dictionary*, 1993)

Unilateral: occurring on one side of the body only.

Vascular: of or relating to a blood vessel. (ref: *The New Shorter Oxford Dictionary*, 1993)

Yin Tuina: A gentle, non-invasive bodywork practised for over 5000 years in China. 'Tuina' means 'push-grasp' in English, while 'Yin' means 'calming or gentle'. 'Yin Tuina' may also be called 'Child Tuina', a gentle, safe and painless therapeutic tool.

APPENDIX 1

Did I Really Have Parkinson's Disease?

This is a question often asked since my recovery. Conservative Western medical wisdom says that nobody gets better if they have Parkinson's disease because they (our Western doctors and scientists) don't have a 'cure'. Therefore, if I recovered, I can't have truly had Parkinson's disease. Complex isn't it?

Actually, it simply needs us to accept that 'cure' is a concept established in Western medical culture, while 'recovery' has been accepted as a real and powerful concept for thousands of years. People recover from all sorts of 'incurable' disorders. When Petrea King and Ian Gawler recovered from their leukemia and cancer, after being told their disorder was 'incurable' and that they would definitely die, many doctors doubted the diagnosis. It has taken over twenty years for these people to be accepted by some (not all) Western oncologists as having wisdom to share with those facing a diagnosis of cancer.

On the other hand, Parkinson's disease is difficult to diagnose because there is no definite test to say 'you have Parkinson's disease'. The disorder is diagnosed from symptoms after all other possibilities have been eliminated.

However, when the set of symptoms is very obvious, and all tests indicate that there is no other cause for those symptoms, we must assume that the person has Parkinson's disease as diagnosed.

My MRI and CT scans showed no other reason for displaying my Parkinson's disease symptoms. I was not taking, and had never taken, any drug that could have caused the symptoms, nor had I been in contact with toxic material that could have caused them. As my symptoms were classically Parkinson's disease and, as I was diagnosed as such by three doctors and several complementary therapists, we must accept, I believe, that the diagnosis of Parkinson's disease was correct.

My symptoms as at early August 1995

- Muscular rigidity in neck, shoulders, back – bilateral but predominantly right side.
- Pain in neck shoulders and back – bilateral but worse on right side.
- Tremor at rest with 'pill rolling' – head and hands – bilateral but worse right side.
- Right shoulder largely immobile – my arm did not swing when I walked and I was unable to use the arm properly even for simple tasks.
- Right leg dragged when walking.
- Right side of face 'frozen' – it did not respond when I smiled or changed expression; I tended to speak from the left side of my mouth.
- Incoherent and/or stammering speech at a low level. However, I could sing quite coherently.
- Ataxia.
- Great fatigue which fluctuated to a small degree with blood sugar levels. I felt as if I was constantly trying to walk against the current in chest high water.
- Weakness in most muscles.
- Intermittent and fluctuating tachycardia/bradycardia/arrhythmia.
- Great difficulty in turning over in bed and I had to roll out of bed in the morning, then pull myself upright using the bed or chair.

- Simple tasks such as dressing became very slow, unco-ordinated and confusing.
- Drowsiness.
- My writing had become smaller and less legible, often degenerating to an almost illegible scrawl running off the line.
- Festinating walk with a widened gait.
- Difficulty in initiating actions, eg. rising from a chair, starting to walk, opening a cupboard.
- Elevated large toes.
- Clawed small toes.
- Poor coordination – eg. couldn't catch.
- Inability to carry out two simple tasks at once – eg. walk and open a bottle.
- 'Freezing' – I used tricks to turn corners, open doors, etc.
- Clumsiness and tendency to drop things.
- Dizzy spells, disorientation and 'absences'.
- My judgement of speed and distance was poor so I had difficulty crossing roads. Driving was risky but the only feasible means of transport.
- Twitching and spasms when relaxed – eg. in bed.
- Intermittent back spasm.
- Reduced visual acuity – I had great difficulty reading newspapers for instance.
- Dyspnea, especially when speaking or at rest.
- Appetite fluctuations without apparent cause.
- Dysphagia – especially with cold drinks.
- Gastric reflux.
- Loss of libido and/or impotence.
- Enuresis.
- Lowered core temperature – I felt the cold much more than I used to.
- Tinnitus, bilateral in my skull well above the ears.

Aqua Hydration Formulas

What's in the Aquas?

The Aqua Hydration Formulas incorporate the principle of synergy; the components of each formula work synergistically.

Each of the Aqua Hydration Formulas contains phyto-homeopathics of Hydrastis Canadensis (Golden Seal), Ulmus fulva (Slippery Elm) and Smilax ornata (Sarsparilla). In addition, phytohomeopathics, herbal extracts and flower essences tailor each of the four formulas for specific roles in male and female bodies.

FEMALE AQUA AM
Extract of Vanilla 1:2
Homeopathics:
  Hydrastis Canadensis 30C
  Ulmus fulva 30C
  Smilax ornate 30C
Bach Flower Essences
Sodium Chloride

MALE AQUA AM
Extract of Vanilla 1:2
Homeopathics:
  Hydrastis Canadensis 30C
  Ulmus fulva 30C
  Smilax ornate 30C
  Opuntia vulgaris 12×
Bach Flower Essences

FEMALE AQUA PM
Extract of Echinacea angustafolia 1:1
Homeopathics:
  Hydrastis Canadensis 11×
  Ulmus fulva 11×
  Smilax ornate 11×
Bach Flower Essences

MALE AQUA PM
Micelized a-Tocopheral
Lavender essential oil
Homeopathics:
  Hydrastis Canadensis 30C
  Ulmus fulva 30C
  Smilax ornate 30C
  Micelized a-Tocopheral 10C
  Iodum 12x
Bach Flower Essences
Sodium Chloride

Source: <www.hydration.org>